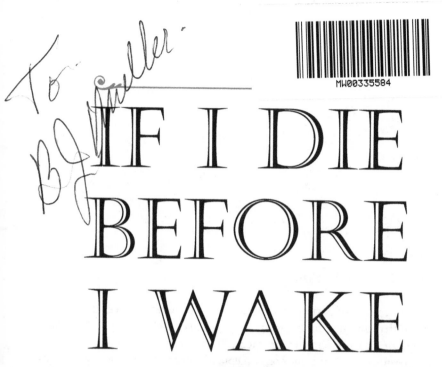

IF I DIE BEFORE I WAKE

A CAREGIVER'S JOURNEY

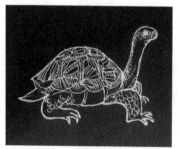

ELI SHAW

Photography on the cover: Stained Glass window by Robert Eli Kershaw Jr.
Photo of author on the back cover by Walter Ward
The artwork behind the author by Paul D

Printed in the United States of America.

Library of Congress Control Number: 2019937678

ISBN   Paperback   978-1-64361-627-8
              Hardback   978-1-64361-628-5
              eBook   978-1-64361-629-2

Westwood Books Publishing LLC
11416 SW Aventino Drive
Port Saint Lucie, FL 34987

www.westwoodbookspublishing.com

DEDICATION

To my family, friends here in the US, and from all over the world, many of whom are mentioned in this book, my mentors who are too many to name, my son Homer, my grandchildren Jamyah and Samueli who I hope will continue my legacy, and to all the students, some of whom are named in this book, you have taught me 100 times more than I could teach you. I also want to thank two of my creative mentors, Aron Martineau and Walt Ward. Katrina, who pushed me when I needed to be pushed and Alex and Bogdan who pulled me out of writer's block. A big thanks to Ed Dunn and Polly Smith for helping me in a pinch and especially to Billie Sue Desrosiers, Editor Extraordinaire. I hope that our relationship as author and reader, will help inspire your relationships with friends, mentors, family, co-workers, to be part of the legacy you leave.

Thank you

TABLE OF CONTENTS

NEED TO KNOW

The first thing you need to know about this book is that at the end of the book some pages are empty. These pages are important because here you can put your thoughts and *ah ha* moments in the book or things you have questions about. I would love to see your thoughts sometime and get inspired by your inspiring moments and if that is not possible, share them with people you love and know.

One of the programs I helped initiate was the Opiate Response Team in one of the local towns in Vermont where I lived for 25 years. I lost several people in my life to pills and heroin. I'm also aware of many young people who are headed that way. When I first approached the Select Board, I told them I'd had enough and need to speak out until something is done. I was assured that we could talk about it and get something going. As time went on with the team, I noticed we were always talking about what we had to offer. The team was comprised of a representative from every part of the community, hospitals, police, schools, retail, churches and organizations. What we missed out doing was setting things up so we could listen first. I was upset at one of the meetings that each group was sharing what they could present to us in the way of services and at times claiming that their way was the best. What we needed to do was listen, not judge and assess what we find. Then we could make decisions as to what would work. The information we were going to give the community can be attained by Google search.

The reason I brought this up is that most of the things in this book are my opinions, points of view, or experiences. I have come to realize that when we post a status on Facebook, we are opening the floodgates to judgment. My purpose for this book is to share what I have experienced, and that is it. I do not like judgemental criticism or comments that are of a demeaning nature as that will be your own opinion and point of view. I would like to see what your thoughts are if they are in a progressive manner or are constructive criticism. If it is just to bash me or the book, keep it to yourself. We are living in a time where we are in a civil war in the form of words. This will only delay good things that can happen or take time away from our lives that are too short as it is. You are welcome to share your thoughts or experiences on my Facebook page or website. I have a cup I use for my morning coffee that someone gave me who knew me well. It says, "This is my opinion, and only I know what it is worth."

The reason why I hold importance to your written thoughts and opinions is that, for me, it is a form of legacy – something I experienced when I found a book my great-grandfather owned. At the back of his book, there were many pages and pieces of paper stuck in the back sleeve of the cover. I began to understand what he wrote. To my astonishment, he became more real, more human and shared any of the beliefs I had about good and evil. He shared his love for helping people and doing what he believed is right. I realized that he, through his scribbles and thoughts at the end of the book, spanned many generations. Even though I never met him, I feel I know him or at least he is a part of me through his notes. His footprint of thoughts reached out far beyond what he could have imagined. It reminds me of the prose poem "Desiderata" by Max Ehrmann. He was an American writer, unknown in his time and has left a legacy that has reached around the world. He wrote this in 1927, and yet it was not widely known until it was used in 1971 – 72 in recordings and put to music.

So, as you continue reading, please feel free to scribble your notes and thoughts at the back of this book. It could be part of your legacy that you may leave to your family and friends or the world.

PREFACE

This book is part of a journey I have been on while not being aware I was on it. I started writing this book after losing my best friend to complications from HIV/AIDS. The same year I lost my Dad and my 90-year-old neighbor. That event was so powerful, I had no idea that because of my prior knowledge of the compassionate life skills of *Caregiving*, it would save me from the insanity that was going on. I have experienced many deaths of friends and loved ones and have come to accept it as a peculiar phenomenon as one of the two miracles that are still mysteries, the other being Birth. I am not talking about violent death; I am talking about the peaceful passage between dimensions as we as humans have created, mostly to comfort us and make the transition understandable.

As a Caregiver, from my first encounter with my childhood friend with Down Syndrome who got bullied to the present, I have always needed to be the change I wanted to see. There is a plaque on my door with that statement to remind me every time I enter my home. Whenever I saw injustice, I always needed to respond with whatever tools I had. Life experiences have been good to me, and I am blessed to have lived the life I have lived. My grandfather told me that if I ever saw an opportunity or a challenge, I should look at it, digest it and spit it out. If it still looks good, do it, because if I do it, it will be apparent whether I succeeded or not, and if I don't, I would never understand. I mentioned this story to a former prisoner of war who had escaped. He told me, that was precisely why he felt he had to make that choice, to go or no. This book is the result of many years of experiencing or experimenting with legacy, caregiving, passion, goals and the need to explore. I hope that if you decide to read it, you can take something positive from it. Life is an education with thousands of teachers. I have tried to be successful with a caring and compassionate nature. So, if you think I am going to write this book as a "how to" or "FYI about AIDS" you are only partially right. This book is about the journey and not in chronological order.

Enjoy my journey and may yours be as enjoyable.

Eli Shaw

A TEMPORARY ASSIGNMENT

Many of our experiences as a Caregiver are only temporary assignments. For the nurse in a hospital, it will only last as long as the patient is there. A doctor usually is only seen for a short time, and the rest of his time he spends checking charts and papers. When a person in the family is ill, it is usually a family member who cares for them and only until he or she gets well or dies. School teachers will only have kids for a year, and then a new group comes in. But for some of us, it can last much longer. I for one have spent twenty-two years with one person as a CPA watching him grow up, but in the end, one of us has to give in or die. Everything we do as a society has something to do with giving care to some degree and outside of all these examples is one main thought - life is a temporary assignment. I learned that at a very young age and it has led me to live my life knowing that someday I will also die, so as long as I am here, I want to do as much as I can. It has brought many people to think that I am self-centered, egotistical, self-absorbing and vain when I only want to experience as much as possible and meet as many people as I can. It is like going to an amusement park for two hours. I want to hit every ride and get as much food as I can while I am there. In doing so, I have lived an amazing life. I have visited many countries, founded a camp, was a photographer, an artist and before I lost my finger, a guitarist. I worked in the school system, worked with the homeless, drug addicts, people with HIV, theatre on Broadway, group homes for the handicapped, elderly and troubled kids and a host of other jobs in retail, industry, and caregiving. Now I am trying my hand at being an author.

When I first decided to write this book in 1992, I had a lot of reservations. AIDS discrimination was one, and in some respects still is. Such a controversial subject. Also, AIDS in the 80s through the 90s, was a death sentence. I was afraid of the discrimination I had seen during the time I was Mark's Caregiver. Mark, a fantastic person in his own respect, was a friend and my roommate for over ten years. We both knew people who were HIV positive, given the venue of employment we were in (retail and theater) and some who had full-blown AIDS. They were coworkers, neighbors, and family friends. I have always thought I was lucky to not have had a family member who was infected. Some were married with kids, some gay and many were just nondescript as far as their lifestyle was concerned. This didn't seem to be a problem at the beginning of our friendship but our ignorance kept us, as it did many others, at a safe distance, or so we thought. Our ignorance can also be added to the list of our many fears. I was more concerned when I read in the newspaper of AIDS discrimination from family members, friends, as well as strangers.

In many cases, I saw instances of violence in the news. At one point, the effects of the community response to AIDS became up close and personal. A co-worker had been beaten because he was HIV positive and his brother, mistaken for his lover was also beaten and later found dead. Even with this being so close, I felt I was at a safe distance. "This only happens to others," I would say. Our fears were confirmed in 1989 when Mark came home with the news that would change both of our lives. It was the news that he was diagnosed HIV positive. He was told that with good eating habits and a good exercise regime along with a good regiment of meds he should be able to live a long life. I questioned this but to not upset Mark, I kept it to myself.

As time went on, we found we were fortunate not to have encountered many situations where discrimination was involved. Only the common fears caused by ignorance would show up, something we could usually handle. We were also white and lived in a suburb of New York City where we could become quite invisible if we wanted to. Sometimes this became an unfortunate thing as it sheltered us from some of the many realities out there concerning AIDS. Much of the "handling" of our concerns, though done in silence, was in the form of looking the other way and carefully screening who we told and who we hung out with. It is sad that we had to stoop to this level of self-preservation, but the situation I found myself in became more and more a matter of survival. He was HIV positive. I was his best friend, roommate and now a Caregiver. Would I be labeled too or would people take us for who we were? I could only imagine what it must be like for those who lived in more deprived areas where health care was limited, and customs of some cultures would rule them out of their social world, or just not be able to tolerate this kind of illness well.

Since Mark's death in 1992, I have been a witness to the problems and frustrations of many who have gone through, and are still going through, the discrimination related to this non-discriminating disease. This is mainly because of ignorance but also because it shakes the foundations of some of the norms of our society. And yes, I said non-discriminating. This Virus, as if it were a lurking demon, does not care who it attacks, or when. It threatens to mutate even more as we look for new cures and hope.

In this society when we see something we don't understand, it becomes a threat and causes us to fear and discriminate against those who might be involved. This has become a truth again with the fear of the Muslim community in the wake of ISIS. We tend to use demeaning remarks and acts against people, and this can lead to low self-esteem and distancing between families, friends, and associates. This thing we call discrimination has gone as far as causing total alienation of these groups, and has been known to be a reason for suicide. At this point, for Mark and me, an alternate plan of action would become necessary for survival, meaning we could have decided who to talk to and how to react to some scenarios. I guess I could have walked away from the situation I found myself in, but Mark was my friend and walking away was just not an option to me.

I used to wonder how long it will take before we begin to educate each other and fight ignorance. I say "used to wonder" but looking at the pandemic in Africa and the ignorance and many times violence that is going on there, I am still wondering.

One of the "ah-ha" moments came during a profound period of my life. This "ah ha" was the realization that for most of my life I have been a Caregiver in one form or another. I also realized that this was all part of a fantastic journey that has not ended, even to this day.

If writing this book and you're reading it, helps even one person get through this or any pandemic or the care of a friend, family member or patient, no matter what the illness or affliction, with as much sanity, dignity and love as I have found, then I am a success. In any situation concerning the illness of a loved one, educating yourself through all the resources available in the community about discrimination or social justice, from libraries to support groups, computers, and educational institutions is important. I sometimes find myself sort of on autopilot and don't think about taking care of myself or how I am doing until someone asks, "How are you doing?". My usual response is, "I am usually fine until someone asks me how I am." Or I say, "I think I am fine, no one has told me differently, so I guess I am fine." Then I must look and see how I really am. This book has become my own personal how am I.

Each of us must deal with everything in very different ways. This again depends on our past experiences, our culture, and education or knowledge at that time. This can change at any moment as we are always growing, learning and experiencing new things. I have found that if I can allow others to go through the process of healing in their own way, I can get through this healing or moment OK also. The key to success is like a recipe. The ingredients are a combination of love, trust, caring and a lot of common sense. If you wouldn't want to be mistreated, don't mistreat others.

In writing this book, I have been able to heal by revealing my experiences as a Caregiver, friend and loved one. It has also helped me to consciously reflect on my decisions with overwhelming satisfaction because I had done what I had done and it was OK. We all learn from our experiences. Whether we choose to accept what we learn and use this knowledge as a tool, is totally up to the individual. My life has changed for the better as I have chosen to use this knowledge to live a more purposeful and fulfilling life. My love for life and all it has to offer, whether hidden or in plain sight, is as vibrant and clear as when I was a child. I have found beauty and peace in sunsets, flowers, people of all origins, the environment and all the things I had taken for granted. Every day becomes a new adventure, full of miracles. I have even found ways to embrace the pessimist in myself and others.

I guess I must sound a little "light in the head" about this but I think that comes with coming to terms with who I am, my experiences and my mortality, as I have had to deal with death as a part of life more times than I want to say. The saying "Life is a temporary assignment" rings true more than ever now. The opportunity to be a witness to life's miracles, give care unselfishly and witness death as one of those miracles, has not only given me hope but has raised enough questions to answer, to last a lifetime. When I am in the role of Caregiver, I am always questioning things, and sometimes the answer resembles a "why me" question. But I found that when the welfare of someone else is in your hands, and the person cannot do things for themselves, I just do what I have to and try not to question things too much or lose the ability I have to preserve and respect that person's dignity or independence. Then, when I am alone, I bitch and moan to myself. Sometimes this is when I get the answers I need and the strength to continue. "It's not about me," I have to tell myself, and that usually does the trick.

When it comes to the subject of dying, I have witnessed so much by now that I have resigned myself to the fact that it may just be just another miracle of life with all its mystery and pain.

In my experiences with the educational system, as a Para Educator and one on one in several situations, I have gotten to know the students well. In most cases, I had to figure out the best way to keep them in school. I also try to help them in the learning process which can be so difficult when their lives outside the school environment can be horrific. The school can become a safe haven at times, and if they can find some reasonable safety there with the people they answer to, it can be a lifesaver. There are so many kids out there and not enough good souls or money to make this system function successfully in my opinion.

Then there is the situation of mental health which has been in the news with all the school shootings and the gun laws being attacked. It is such a fine line between seeing someone do something unusual and asking for a mental health assessment and just being eccentric and harmless. It is indeed a tough one. Yet we have some of the most innovative programs for disabilities and mental health. The school systems are squeezed to death at times from regulation, recording and the financial crisis. Our taxes pay for a lot of it and when people see where it is distributed it can be a monumental task running successfully enough to not affect the clients. That goes for the educational institutions also.

I hope you enjoy reading my book and if it helps you in any way, I hope you can find the time to share it and your own experiences with caregiving, illness or death in any sense with someone you care about or who cares about you. We can't fight these questions and concerns alone. The process can look like the enemy. So, the only thing I can suggest is to find ways to lighten the load.

Thank you for the time you will spend, and I hope you will feel it will have been well spent.

Taking Things for Granted

In any situation after spending so much time with someone, we as humans have the possibility of taking this person, and situations we find ourselves in with them, for granted. This person could be a mother, father, wife, husband, lover, sister, brother or friend. Also, situations, events, and life-changing cycles can, and are eventually taken for granted as we get used to their presence in our lives. For me, taking relationships for granted was like Christmas day when I was a child. Those first glimpses of toys and brightly colored boxes with shimmering bows under the tree became so special and unique. I wanted to hold on to it forever. All of my attention was focused on my new-found treasures. I would hurry to the base of the tree and tear open those blocks of glitter and magic that was so carefully created the night before to camouflage the reality of my recent dreams and wishes, subliminally suggested to my elders throughout the past year.

In most cases, the moment would last a few hours, usually until everyone had received theirs as I patiently waited out of sheer respect. Yet there was always that tiny glimmer of hope that there might be one more for me. Sometimes the excitement would continue for a day. Occasionally I would be fortunate enough to experience it for several days. However, there always comes that moment when I would look at the tree with all the toys around it except for that special one I had carefully chosen and saw that there were no children or adults to be seen. The moment was over. Just a memory was left.

I have, in the past, taken for granted those moments of joy, specialness, sense of love and belonging and sharing as if I can recapture it at any given moment. This seems to be what many of us do in our relationships. I know, I have done this. Yet I have known people who have found a way to savor these moments, even though they may be few and far between. This act of taking things for granted is typical and will probably continue to be a routine encounter as long as we live. We take for granted that the sun will come up each morning, so we sleep in and miss the sunrise. If there ever came a time when we knew it was going to be the last time, we would see the sun forever, we would probably take in all the rays we could before it went away.

There will be times in our lives when we will come to realize how special we and the people and things that surround us are. Looking back at my time with Mark, I remember how special it was the day we both got caught in the worst rainstorm I had seen. Yet we decided to just keep walking and enjoy the experiences as everyone rushed around us. We began to realize how close our friendship, and sharing that went with it, was. I am sure you can look back at some crazy time you shared with a friend or relative that seems to come up in conversations now and then as, "remember the time we . . .". Even the disagreements we had that would send us crashing into a wall of reality were vital because they weeded out the unwanted parts of our friendship.

Look closely at your friendships. See how they came about or developed over the years. Notice how unique certain important parts of your experiences were. Look at the hard times and how they may have tightened up the loose ends of the friendship that you may now take for granted.

The experiences you will read about in this book could relate to anyone. If you have consciously taken a breath, been startled at the barking of a dog or a loud noise, been exhilarated after a cool plunge in a cold clear pond, been overcome with joy at the meeting of a friend not seen for some time and anyone who has experienced the birth of their child, death of a loved one, illness, kindness, sadness, anger, confusion or torment. This is not a "cure-all book" or a "claim to have the answers book." It is a book about my journey through my eyes.

Now take a few minutes, look around you and pick ten simple things that you might have taken for granted. My ten things were water, the sun, my van, my sister and two brothers, my friends far and near, electricity, my health, the telephone, the gas station and my sight which is vitally important to me being that I am also a photographer. In 2007, I discovered I have glaucoma which raised my awareness that I took sight for granted for so long. Now think what it might be like to go without some of them. In the case of my sister and two brothers, what it would be like if I needed their help and they were not there? On the subject of gas, have you ever been on a highway when all of a sudden you look at your gas gage and discover it was a hair above empty, and you don't know where the next gas station is? Does panic ring a bell? Taking something for granted means you expect it will be there when you need it. When it isn't, you feel at a loss as well as so many other emotions, usually anger at yourself for allowing it to happen.

Can you see what I mean about taking life and all its components for granted? Certainly, we can't go around thinking this way all the time. But as you read this book keep in mind how we do take things for granted. I hope that you may want to look at life, people, things and all their components with a little more respect and compassion. If you are a Caregiver, you may understand what I mean. Also, allow yourself the opportunity to look at stress and its causes and see if you could do something to lessen it. I sometimes take stress for granted and stress can be a significant factor in the success or failure of our caregiving. As I now still take stress for granted, I see how it affects my physical and mental life. My friend, who is a Psychologist and at times my guru, has made me well aware that I am high maintenance. I did not understand what that meant in the beginning and still have trouble making myself aware of this concept. One of her latest responses to a message was, "Call it squelching the have to's of aliveness. You seem to still need to be the hamster on his wheel. There is nothing wrong with you. I repeat, NADA wrong. You just take yourself for granted like most people I encounter when they're suffering physical maladies." So, you see it is still happening to me, taking myself for granted.

I guess I could go on forever, as my friends say I will do from time to time. However, there is just one more thing I would like to mention. This book is also about looking at things in your life that may not be needed and are like fallen trees on the road to where you are going. The experiences I am about to share made me aware of all the "stuff" in my life, good and bad. A good analogy for me is when a drain gets clogged, it interrupts the flow. I have created my fair share of clogs and continue to do so.

Many times, I hesitate to do something about my stuff or "fallen trees" or a situation thinking that it is not as important as it might be or I can put off attending to it until another time. When I might be forced to go in a different direction in life for whatever reason, it sometimes gives me a chance to see the things I don't need and act on them. If you have ever been terminated from a job, you know what I mean. In a job where there is a lot of stress, you may think you need to take the aggravation of dealing with the stress. Suddenly the job isn't there. The need to take the aggravation isn't there, and we have a learning experience. This happened to me at a job I thought was the best job I had ever had. It had theatre, antiques, volunteers, education, retail and I was the manager. I received so much positive reinforcement about what I was doing, I thought I would never leave. After about a year, I was taken out to lunch and was thanked for all I had done. Then out of nowhere, I was told they had to let me go as they needed to downsize. WOW! I had overcome all the aggravation the job had and made it my own, and suddenly it was not there anymore. Some situations are more difficult than others. When we are in the position of Caregiver, there may be many things we must look at, as I did. I looked at the amount of time I spent on the phone and with whom. Listening to what is being said, how important it was to me and whether I was neglecting something or someone and taking something or someone for granted became important.

I still take a lot of things for granted. The difference is, I know when I do. This also presents me with the opportunity to do something about it.

All I ask of you is to take what works for you. Learn from the experiences I am sharing with you. Judge only yourself and things closely related to you. Don't judge yourself too harshly and live your life as if it were only a temporary assignment, an important one.

Thank you and Peace.

IF I DIE BEFORE I WAKE

The original title of this book was "Caring for Mark." I later realized that this was more than just caring for one individual. It was a journey. The title of this chapter became my second choice. Mark would frequently say, "If I die before I wake up, make sure you get everything in order," and he would proceed to give me a list of things I had to do.

Several more chapters were written before I realized that again the journey became the focal point. It was a journey that began many years ago and has brought me to this place. Everything else was all a part of this journey I was on. Lately, I am finding that it has become a life long journey and has encompassed everything I do. Like any ailment or addiction, I need to admit it, truly admit it myself to do anything about it.

To some of you who have picked up this book, the story will be familiar. Familiar, not only in an environment where the AIDS virus is the focus, but also if you who have gone through any caregiving situation where a person being cared for is at a terminal stage. Also working with people who find they may not be able to walk again or have lost use of some of their senses can have the same problems and earmarks of someone who is facing death. This story is more about the caregiving side of it. This story is only one of the millions of stories with a similar substance, and unfortunately, there will be millions more to come. I have dedicated a lot of this book to caregiving connected with HIV/AIDS mainly because a lot of my "ah ha's" about life as a Caregiver came about during my caregiving experiences with people who were HIV positive. One of the key components of success is to not become the victim as I did and still do. At least now I know when I do this which is half the battle.

At a conference in 1994, the prediction was made that by the year 2000 more than 40,000,000 people will have been infected worldwide. That was a good guess as since the beginning of the epidemic, 75,000,000 have been infected to date (2019) worldwide. Because of the advances in medicine, the death rate has gone down but the infection rate has gone up. In 2017, approximately 39.9 million people are presently living with the virus worldwide. 43% of that group are women. In 2017 940,000 died in that year alone. Because so many people died in the early years who were never counted for reasons of shame and confidentiality, I believe there can never be an accurate count. With the rise in Diabetes related illnesses, drug addiction, Alzheimer's and dementia, Cancer, Parkinson's, and so many others and the deaths that go with them, the caregiving experience and industry will expand, grow and intensify also. Because we have not yet found a cure for all of these, the march goes on. Yes, we are getting better at not ignoring it all for economic, social, cultural and religious reasons as much as we used to but we have a long way to go.

My story is probably not any worse nor better than any of yours. Since July 1992 when Mark, died, I have been meeting people who were Caregivers as well as people who were part of this growing population with terminal illnesses. In doing so, I have found that many people go through this process of caring, illness, and loss, without knowing where to go for help and support or if there was any help out there at all. Also, because it is such an exhausting process with people putting their routinely normal lives on hold so to speak, we tend to close the door on opportunities. When this happens we put our routine or book of life on the shelf for a while as we try to deal with the daily routines introduced to us by whomever we are caring for and whatever they have. Later when circumstances change for whatever reason, we find ourselves picking up the pieces of our lives and trying to continue where we left off.

When we put our book of life on the shelf, we tend to leave out our experience of caregiving, AIDS, cancer, illness, fear, exhaustion and loss. By loss, I also mean the loss of one's "self." This presents another problem. This personal library is not available to the public, and we tend to guard it carefully. Those who follow have no more to go on than the ones who came before. This has changed since the 90s, but it could be better. I do admit that lately more and more books and talk shows, the Caregiver's networks on social media (such as Facebook with The Caregivers Space, and Caregivers Hub) and courses in school are taking a stand and talking more about all of this. I believe we have come to a place in time where, while it won't be any easier, we will have more knowledge to work with. I don't mean that everyone should write a book, or write a diary, although it seems that there are books out there on everything, I mean share your experiences and the knowledge you gain.

We should be able to talk about the experience with others. Many of us, myself included, don't talk about it out of concern or fear that they would be bringing up bad or unpleasant memories and the possibility of breaching the confidentiality of the ones being cared for. The fear of being judged can become an issue which was my biggest fear for a long time and still is to some extent with today's political happenings. "What will they think of me" becomes a question we all can relate to. In our society, we tend to judge and be judged all through our lives. From learning how to fit in while in elementary school to sitting in an interview for a college or a job, we are always being judged.

For many years after World War II, people held in the memory of the horrors which occurred in all parts of the world. Many died with these memories and were never healed. Many would not share because of the pain of remembering, while others felt they would be judged or labeled if they did. For some, it wasn't until someone asked them about it many times that they opened their "book" to the world. It is this act of courage that can begin the healing process and give people the sense that they are not alone.

Doing this presented the opportunity to open up and share their pain, joy, hate, and anger with others. This process is one used in support groups all over the world and one I use in healing myself as I try to find my way back to a normal and somewhat stable existence. Sharing with friends was hard at times because we all can judge others, even our friends. This fear of being judged kept me silent for a while until I began to write down what I went through. Until I was able to see, in front of me, the journey I had taken and the pain I had experienced, I was but a small piece of the larger puzzle that didn't seem to make a difference. I have gone through several types of psychotherapy in the past, some helped, and some made me worse and compromised my blood pressure, stress and health until I was able to learn how to let it go. I still am high maintenance, but I am beginning to understand that more. It affects everything I do but I still resist being judged even if it is for my own good.

In many cases, I found that getting help means being told many times that I was not normal or whole. That can suck - no, that does suck. Deep inside I have always been happy with who I am and what I have done until someone tells me I am not, and I need to change or get better. But that is just me.

I am sure others will have their opinion about that. I always wonder where that comes from. Feeling like a subject that someone can study and judge is not something I enjoy. However, that said, I have always been able to learn from what and how people judge me.

My journey ranged from working with the disabled, kids with cancer, TBI and mental health, AIDS and diabetes, which was the one that closed my book for a long time. It caused writer's block for a period of time. I feared and still fear what people will think or how they will treat me. I have always felt that if you give out a lot of information it can be used as ammunition by others against you or to "help" you get better. Scandals in the technological world is a good example of letting out too much information and not knowing how it will be used against you.

I recently experienced the suicide of a friend. Because I worked with the kids in his family, and the alienation I experienced from the community and friends, was tragic. She finally decided to move out of the town where she was very well known and respected until that time. There was more to this story. The opinions of some of the community, who without full knowledge ran with it with a vengeance. Most of the pain was directed toward the mom and the daughter who was attending the local school. Also, because I was part of the family structure working with their son with a disability some of the finger-pointing was directed toward me. Working in the school system gave me a glimpse of what was being said out there. Most of what I heard from the kids had to have come from something they heard at the dinner table or in the community. Not getting the support from some of the faculty gave me a window into how they felt. I now know, fear of being judged unjustly goes a long way. As you can imagine, this is something that has affected me greatly.

Getting back to the subject of the chapter at hand, I began to share my experiences as a Caregiver to others and found I was not alone. As I would share, they would in turn share that they too had taken the roller coaster ride which most Caregivers experience as well. We began to compare notes. I found myself not criticizing myself as much for the silly things I did or thought while going through the process of giving care but allowing forgiveness and compassion which in turn, for me, speeded up the healing process.

Being angry became a regular event, and at times I wondered if I should bother getting mad as I was not sure who or what to direct my anger towards. However, angry I did get. Yet, by allowing myself to be angry at the pandemic and the people who were making it difficult for me and millions of others, I was able to forgive them more freely, as well as myself, for getting angry. Ignorance, another sore spot, became an obsession with me and a reason for me to get fired up. My usual response was a resounding and furious "How can you not know that?" or "What is going on?" or "You are so ignorant."

As I was so focused on everyone else's ignorance, I became blind of my own ignorance until I began seeing glimpses of the ignorance I was harboring and protecting like it was an injured kitten. I was finding reasons why it was ok to be ignorant as if it would keep me safe or something. I became more judgmental of myself than I used to be with others which was a painful awakening for me. I had to change that. One day, as I was watching a program on TV something was said that put a light on what ignorance was. To this day I cannot remember what was said, but it helped me begin to look at the ignorance as the beginning of knowledge rather than the end of a conversation or the beginning of a conflict. I finally came to the realization which would change the way I thought about ignorance in so many ways. That revelation was that we are all ignorant of everything at some point in our lives and once we understand this, we can begin to know. Everything we do and know we had to learn except for breathing, etc.

Most of my ability to learn and survive came from my upbringing. That is where this journey began. I grew up in a very liberal family. We had our rules and chores, but we were free to explore and learn. One of my parents' rules was to be mindful of the needs of others which was later reinforced in the church in the form of a prayer which I heard each Sunday by Rev. Ulrich. The words, "Keep us ever mindful of the needs of others through Christ our Lord, Amen" stuck with me. If something or someone was different, my parents encouraged me to learn to understand the situation or person before making any judgments and then be cautious about those judgments. In the family environment, I felt safe and protected. Outside the family, there was the fear of being judged. The fashion or trend of the popular kids was straight hair, and I had a curly top. I may have had the first afro. The nickname, Curley or "n" knots was so upsetting to me as a young kid.

Seeing how others were treated and judged made me wonder what people thought of me and if I was being misjudged. I often wondered if that was true for everyone. In grammar school and especially junior and senior high school, I was particularly sensitive and on my guard. The sixties rebellion was an example of people wanting to understand but society putting a halt on the process. Being judgmental also went hand in hand with racism, religion and political opinion.

Over 60 years have passed and we are still doing it, being judgmental that is, with Arabic nations, AIDS and the fact that in 2008, we didn't just elect a president, we elected a black president and the fact that we say a black president shows me that racism is still in play. Even though he is half black and half white, we still call him black. How can we call him black? Why not white or black and white. Or better yet, let's just call him president. None of the white presidents had emphasis by the society on being white. Concerning AIDS, cancer, diabetes, Alzheimer's and all the other ailments we do not fully understand, I feel just as angry now about the judgments we place on these ills, as I did then, but I am now more open to listen and understand and then speak out. We all pass judgments, and yes, some of them hurt and maim others. Whether it is intentional or not or a tool to raise ourselves to a higher level, as we loom over our victims as in the incident at Abu ghraib Prison or feel we can heal others if they do it our way, it is still a human trait we will always have. Most of the time it is done very quietly, and the victim may or may not know it has happened.

A friend of mine asked why I was writing this book. I had to look deep, and I must say, some reasons are personal as far as healing and just getting it out of my system. Some reasons are professional, but I also wanted to just see if I could do it. The main reason comes from the caring side of me where I want others to have the opportunity to see where they may have also been and know they are not alone in this conversation. Also, know that there are many support groups for families and friends who have lost someone or are possibly caring for someone with cancer, AIDS, the elderly, Alzheimer's or an accident victim. It is not easy to share in a world not ready to receive what you have to share without being judged. I have been accused of being a good giver but a bad receiver. It is true, after looking at that accusation closer. Something I guess I must work on. As you can see, writing this book is becoming a journey of discovery for me. Mostly discovering why the hell I am doing it.

Several years ago, a former student of mine Brian Griffin had an accident. Before the accident, he was a wild one in ways and lived life like he was going to live forever. The accident left him with a TBI. His life changed forever. When he came out of the hospital, he had to learn how to live again and understand who he was and how he was going to survive. Slowly, he became a calm, inquisitive young man externally. I have been lucky enough to have known him before and after the accident. To be honest, this brief entrance in this book does no justice to this man's transformation and struggles. I have made sure I have seen or talked to him once a week. One thing he told me was that as he was evolving into someone he did not know, people would say things like, "Well you used to do it this way" or "Remember when you used to...." This frustrated him to no end as in many cases he had no memory of it or did not want to remember it. Having that sensitivity as a Caregiver, I had to watch myself as I knew all his antics in school. This young man had such an emotional impact on my life, and I have become closer to him as a friend. He has taught me volumes about life and myself on this journey.

Since my youth, I have been a person who loved to explore new boundaries and writing this book is one. While writing this book, I have worked on another project of mine which I feel needs to be done. I spoke with many people who were HIV positive. I wanted to see if Mark's experience was "normal." While talking to them, I found new energy I hadn't experienced before except with Mark. It was positive energy, no pun intended, that later in his illness, he was too weak to develop. Many of the people I spoke to had a real zest for life and a real need to share more openly but were in fear of being judged or just didn't have a vehicle to do so. With every person I spoke to I got the feeling they needed a platform or a way to get their message out as Mark wished he could have had done.

With my talent as a photographer and my willingness to listen and share, I began a project called "If I Die Before I Wake." It is a collection of photos of people who were HIV positive and a script written by them to the right of the photo. This was a chance for them to say what they had to say without being face to face with so many others. The exhibit has been presented as an exhibit at the Cathedral of St. John the Divine in New York City on Amsterdam Ave and 115th Street among other public events and venues. The impact and differences this show made on people all over the world were evident in the messages left in the guest book. It was something I did not expect. Each visitor had an opportunity to share his or her experience with the show by writing in the guest book on the table. One eye-opening incident was when I set up the exhibit in Brooklyn, NY and a mother of one of the subjects saw her sons' picture and script in the exhibit. Even though I had his signed release, the mother was affected by it. She asked that I take it down. I did remove it in respect to the family and their privacy and safety. I found I had to be open to all of this. The letters I have received and comments left have given me an incentive to continue learning more about a lot of things. This incentive has led me to a sense of joy, change, sincerity, and an affirmation to make a difference daily. A very high maintenance endeavor I am told. There are also scripts from the exhibit in the back of the book.

Like Mark, these people have changed the scope of the rest of their lives whether it be from HIV/AIDS, Cancer or any other illness to a more focused position. This is something we all would like to be able to do, but most of the time we are too busy putting things off for another day.

One of the individuals I had the pleasure of speaking to told me, "you know, life is a hoot." By hoot, she meant funny or wonderful. Coming from someone who most of us would say was "dying with AIDS," this might seem a little strange. After speaking with her for some time, I began to realize she is more alive or aware than most of us will ever be. She said, "It is almost like a train ride or road trip to a place we have never been to before. Most people worry about getting there or work frantically at getting things ready and then miss the scenery. Life to me is just a means to get to a higher place, and there are so many things to see on the way." She was enjoying the people and the scenery. The bumps and potholes were just part of it all. She just hit a big pothole.

When Mark died in 1992, he was 32 years young. Now to someone who is in their teens, 32 can be considered old. I know how I felt at 15.

If I hadn't accomplished everything I wanted to do by 30, I would be a failure. I am now 70. What does that tell you? It is incredible how so many things stay the same even as time goes on or changes.

When he died, I was on the left side of the hospital bed and his mother on the right. I saw his mother with emotions that didn't make sense to her. Her son physically got older and died before she did. It isn't supposed to happen that way. But I also saw a woman who had so much love to give and a son who was receiving it and giving it right back right to the end. Mark was a meticulous person. For example, the day before he died, he was balancing his checkbook. Hey, you never know. In a way, it all made sense and yet it didn't. It would be awhile before I could see how it did. I am still on a journey to understand it all.

The movie "Forrest Gump," shows us an excellent example of this journey and how he dealt with it. When he was running and running and got to a place where he thought was the end of his journey, he put his expectation of ending aside and found another direction to go to continue the journey. In the end, he realized it was always OK to just go home. Even this becomes a part of the journey.

I only hope if you are in a place where you are holding expectations of a finale, you can see another door that can be opened and new worlds can be explored. When we hold on to an ending, we tend to do nothing. When we are doing nothing, we must realize that doing nothing is part of the journey and that it is OK if you let it be OK. But remember the door. I recently experienced this with the loss of that fantastic job. I found the new doors I have been able to open.

Many of my experiences have been eye-openers and learning experiences within the journey. The things I have learned however can be applied to any given situation no matter how small. Look at your journey and all the stops you might have had during it. Hopefully, this book will only be a pit stop on your journey, as it has been for me and an incentive to continue and find new directions. Good luck and thank you for giving me the opportunity to share and for allowing yourself to receive, something I am still in the process of doing.

I think what Mark was saying when he said, "If I die before I wake, make sure this is done", was that it is so important to get things in order so that others do not have to finish up the loose ends. This is something I am desperately working on. Yet I do enjoy my stuff even if it looks cluttered. So, if you die before you wake, what are you leaving undone or to someone else to complete?

IGNORANCE IS BLISS

I moved to College Point, Queens, New York in April of 1981 after taking an offer I couldn't refuse. My roommate and friend Chuck, had taken on a job as a sales rep for a wire and cable company in New York based in North Carolina. He had heard me mention that I had often thought it would be fun to work in New York doing window display and store design for retail companies, something I was good at and had been doing since I was 15 years old.

One evening in Salem, New Hampshire where I was living, Chuck came home with a big grin on his face. I knew something awesome happened. I had just recently lost my mother to a stroke and a heart attack and was also working for a group home for mentally challenged individuals and part-time at a department store as an interior display designer. To say the least, I was in a state of limbo and could have been swayed toward a change with no commitments to anyone except the clients at the group home.

My Mom's death was one of those unfinished business deaths where she went suddenly, and even though we spoke at least two or three times a week, I felt there was a lot left unsaid. I didn't expect her to die so soon. It would be many years before I would feel complete with her death.

Chuck's mood was more of a euphoric high which I attributed to a few drinks he might have had earlier to celebrate something. We sat in the living room and watched TV for a while. Being the methodical thinker and planner that he was, I felt he had something he wanted to tell me. "So, what's up," I said. He hesitated a bit and said, "I'll tell you soon."

I have always hated it when someone approaches a conversation like that, leaving me hanging on a limb. All kinds of things came into my head, and of course, I thought the worst. He got up and walked into his room and shut the door. I was never one to handle very well those situations of silence and not knowing. I usually internalized my feelings, which is precisely what I did.

Think positive, I thought to myself as I proceeded to bed. Pacing back and forth as I undressed, I created every scenario in detail and technicolor in my head, always emphasizing the worst. I finally calmed down and must have fallen asleep after an hour of tossing and turning. Suddenly, I was awakened when the door flew open and Chuck plowed into my room and sat on the edge of my bed. "I got a job in New York and have to leave in a couple of months," he said. "I know you want to go to New York to test your skills and I am going to need someone to set up an apartment while I go to North Carolina for some training." He was never much of a homebody, as I did most of the cooking. I had the design skills, as eclectic as they were, so I said, "you want me to go to New York and set up your apartment and then what? Do I come back and continue my life as it was or stay there with no job and no money to fall back on?"

He laughed and said, "No you can stay there until you get a job. I will help you out as much as I can if I get paid back any money I spend on your stay there. You don't have to make a decision now, but I need to know soon." As you may imagine, my mind began to race. Getting to sleep was no easy task.

While working at the group home for the mentally challenged, I had made a lot of friends. I also had a great relationship with the residents. How was I going to tell them I was leaving and how could I make that transition a smooth one? This should have been easy for me as I have uprooted myself many times before. But this time it was New York City, The Big Apple. This was a scary thought indeed. I spent about a week thinking it over. The residents had pulled me through some rough times during my mother's death, and it was going to be hard to let all of this go. I had done this before, I thought to myself.

However, this time was going to be a test. My life was about to change dramatically. Yet because of my nature to care for others, this change would have some familiarity with it. I would be taking care of Chuck, and that made the transition easier somehow. Working in the group home also gave me a view of caregiving I had never experienced before. It was coupled with a great deal of responsibility and structure which is something in my life I have yet to conquer.

I spoke to my supervisor and a few friends. I asked if they would support me in making this a smooth transition. They all knew this was a move I wanted to make and said to me, "Give it some thought, and we will support you 100% whatever you decide." With that load off my mind, I proceeded to plan my escape so to speak. I had sessions with the residents to make the final decision, and then I could tell Chuck I would go.

That night I came home and began to pack my things. Chuck came home soon after and caught me packing. He just smiled and hugged me and then said, "you will never regret this move."

The move went smoothly. We filled the truck in one evening and were off for the Big Apple. I remember feeling scared and uncertain about the change I was about to make in my life, but I think I had more of a sense of adventure which compensated for the fear. This would be my chance to explore a whole new world. On the way to New York I thought about all the experiences I had with the residents and how, even with their disabilities, they showed me a lot more than I could have ever shown them in the way of letting life happen and making it all work. They will always be in my thoughts. As a Caregiver in the group home, I was someone they all were supposed to look up to and respect, but they taught me that they were also human beings with feelings and dreams. Their abilities outweighed their disabilities. Some were blind, but they taught me how to see. Some were physically disabled, but they taught me how to walk proudly. I can't measure what they taught me. Only one word comes to mind - Priceless.

I had been in New York for only a few months and was beginning to settle down. Jobless, except for my weekend job at the Milk Barn in

College Point where I worked as a Deli Clerk. I got about $50.00 a week. This gave me enough for my train fare into the city and back with a couple of cups of coffee on the side. I would schedule my job interviews at different times so I could have enough time to get from one to the other without public transit as it would save me a few bucks. This taught me a lot about being frugal. It was the first time I had to really look at what I spent wherever I went, and I feel it became an eye-opener for me. To this day I try to remember where I was at that time. Unfortunately, we all forget, and I do forget sometimes and spend too much.

The time I spent in the city also gave me a chance to see what the real New York was like and experience the many cultures and the people that made the city almost a living organism. I remember getting off the train at Grand Central Station. Fascinated by the size of the space and as a true newcomer or tourist would, I kept looking up. Suddenly I went head over heels onto the sidewalk. I had just tripped over one of the homeless men who was laying horizontal over the threshold of the doorway leading out to 42nd Street. Not knowing much about the homeless situation, I leaned over and was about to give the guy a hand. I thought he might be hurt.

Suddenly a man behind me tapped me on the shoulder and said, "You want to help him, right?"

I said, "Yes, he is hurt, isn't he?"

The guy just smiled and pointed down the street toward Lexington Ave. After a brief pause and a deep breath, he leaned over to me and said, "If you help him you will want to help him, and him, and him...."

"Ok," I said. "You made your point." I brushed myself off and reached into my pocket to give the homeless guy a quarter as I didn't have much to offer at that point. Then I headed toward my next interview but this time with a new real fear. I was only a few steps away from being homeless myself. That was something I thought about for a long time after.

This brought back the memory of one of my first experiences in New York just after arriving. I had all my money in a metal box in the back of the trunk of my car and all the portfolios and pictures I had of my experiences with visual merchandising and store design. I had stopped to get something to eat and parked on the side of the building. When I came out, my car and everything I owned that was not in the moving truck we had loaded, was gone. I had nothing, and Chuck was on his way to North Carolina for training. I had no money and no way to get to where I wanted to go. I felt close to being homeless except I had a home, was not sure of the location and my furniture and clothes were there. It was getting late, and I was not sure where to go. I saw a church nearby and found a place in the back of it to sit. While sitting, I fell asleep out of exhaustion. Later that night the pastor came in and saw me there. When he woke me, my first thought was that I was going to be arrested for loitering or something. He assured me I would be ok and heard my story. He offered me a cot in the back office and something to eat. Scared, I took his hospitality and went to sleep hoping I would find my car and possessions untouched. The next morning, I got up to a lot of noise and a lot of people. I rustled myself together and walked up to where the noise was coming from. My first thought was to leave as soon as I could so as not to disturb whatever was going on. What I saw when I got there was a group of men, tattered clothes and unshaven, standing in line.

I went back to where I had been sleeping and looked around for the pastor. Seeing him in his office, I went in and asked him what this place was. He told me it was the neighborhood soup kitchen. Talk about luck. I got to eat and eventually helped in the kitchen for a while that morning. The pastor offered to help me find my apartment and gave me some money to hold me over. It wasn't until many months that I realized how close to being homeless I was. I could have been that guy I tripped over or one of those anonymous faces standing in line for a bite to eat. While there I got to talk to some of the guys. I was amazed to hear some of their stories. Their past lives, as they called it, ranged from executive to bus driver. How they got there made me realize how fragile we are and how just a slip of the pen or loss of a job could catapult us headlong into homelessness. I was lucky to find my car when a friend of mine from New Hampshire called and told me that the police were looking for me to return my car as they found it abandoned on the side of the road. I went to the station, and they told me it would cost about $100 to get it out of the impound. I went down to get it and found that the money and portfolios and some odds and ends were gone, it was out of gas, but it was intact.

Those experiences and a few others were some of the more sobering experiences of my 18 years in New York. I am sure I will always remember them. For some time after, these memories sent shivers up my spine and weakened my knees at the thought that I might become one of the homeless if I didn't get my act together. Talk about an incentive to do well. Yet every time I see a homeless person it reminds me of how lucky I am. I was, and sometimes am only a train fare away from being where they are. My bank account was non-existent at that time, and I had debts to pay back. I have always tried to pay back anyone who lent me a hand. If I could not right away, I would eventually. Now especially with the economy the way it is, I am very aware of what I do and yet I am always willing to help others. I think it is a part of my faith or the astrological effects on my life, as I have recently discovered. I have always believed that if you give what you can afford to give, it will come back to you ten-fold, not so much as money but also in many other ways. I have found this to be a truth in my life in recent times as some people I had helped several years ago have been helping me with the renovation of my house.

As time went on, I was out there diligently looking for a job. Any job. I met so many people in so many situations and began to realize that New York was full of people willing to help in some way. There I was standing on 42nd Street in a second-hand pinstriped suit that Chuck had given to me to get me started. Even though the suit hadn't been cleaned in a while for lack of funds, there I was, looking for a job. I always tried to look my best, or the best I could look.

With so much time on my hands between interviews, I noticed that people in New York love to talk when they are given a chance. Many tell wonderful stories, and with all this time I had, I could afford to listen. I'm sure some of it was a line of bull, but they sounded good. Then I realized that they also love to listen. Not like in New England, where many people I knew were ready to interrupt, trying to out storytell the other. New Yorkers seemed to listen. I found out I could get connections and information about a lot of things I would normally have a hard time acquiring. It was like I was networking in a way, but I did not know I was doing it at the time. Now we rely on our personal computers and iPads to get informed or just find directions, but in 1982, the computer was a long way off.

One of my goals was to become a visual merchandiser, store or set designer, with windows being the easier and more visible option. I had gone to several job agencies but was not getting too far with them. Remember I lost my portfolio and pictures of anything I had done, I was either overqualified or didn't have enough experience in the city. My days were spent walking by hundreds if not thousands of store window displays and always feeling I could do a better job. Such a critic I was.

Back at the apartment having established myself in College Point, Queens, I had a few books by Gene Moore of Tiffany's, who was one of the most famous window designers in one of the most famous stores in the world. Chuck was getting a little frustrated with me not getting a real job as he called it. He sometimes commented that I was not doing enough and the clock was ticking. That was something I was well aware of. I felt he was being unfair putting a lot more stress on me but he was right and, in some ways, it gave me a push to get it done.

One day I had an idea. Sitting in my living room having my morning coffee and worrying about my future, I thought, if I could only contact Mr. Moore of Tiffany's, he might give me some ideas of where to go or better yet, a job. I got the number from the information operator (remember this was the 80s) and made several calls but was not able to connect. I did leave a message that, to my recollection, rambled on about my dilemma. One morning I got a call. It was Mr. Moore. I felt star-struck and humbled. I must have babbled on for a while until finally, he said, "Well why don't you come in and we can have lunch and talk about where you want to get to." Well, if you think that didn't shut me up, think again. I shut up! I don't remember if I said goodbye or not. So much for great first impressions.

I am not sure when my feet hit the ground again, but I do remember meeting him. It was one of those high points in your life you don't forget. In short, his advice to me was to keep dreaming and keep looking and look for something you can love doing. Also, try to land a job you can develop into "YOUR" job, sort of taking ownership of it. I didn't quite understand what that meant, but I do now. He was telling me to look for a job or position that I could mold and develop where I had a lot of control and creativity and could own the job. The other thing he warned me about was to look out for the barracudas, as he called them, and backstabbers or people users. The industry is full of them but there are also many wonderful people and to know the difference is to succeed. I have tried to carry that idea with me in all my jobs. I won't say I succeed all the time, but I carry it with me.

WOW! Talk about a great day. His advice has stuck with me to this day in all aspects of my life. What I learned for myself was that if I put my mind to it, I could do anything I wanted to.

Finally, after several months, I got a job at Swensen's Ice Cream, which was also a restaurant. It was a far cry from designing windows, but it was a job. It was also across from a comedy club and in an area where many creative people lived and hung out. That afternoon I had a few extra bills in my wallet to celebrate, so I went to one of the local bars in the Village (Greenwich Village) where Swensen's was located and had a few brews. It was around that time I had noticed some of my friends I had made in N.Y. were getting quite ill, and it was as if they were growing old at an accelerated rate. I found out later, a couple of them had died.

While sitting at the bar talking to a few of the so-called locals, I noticed a can on the bar with the letters AIDS on it and above it was GMHC (Gay Men's Health Crisis). I asked the bartender what it was for. With a look on his face that said, where have you been hiding, he began to explain to me what AIDS was and how I could get involved in looking for the cure or politically. This was sounding like another cancer campaign or March of Dimes thing, which I tried to support each year if I could. I threw in a few quarters to quiet him and hoped he would go away. I had just given him the coffee money for my morning coffee to wake me up on my next ride into the city. That was a lot of money for me at the time. Yet what I did that day still haunts me. To think that I was that ignorant about AIDS, the epidemic that could wipe out a huge portion of our population, today makes me ill.

A while later some articles were surfacing about HIV/AIDS. I had just lost a friend from a disease that few people knew much about and had heard that the doctor couldn't believe he had died of what he had so quickly. Who knew?

As the years went on, AIDS became a focal point and controversy in many communities. People were handing out literature about this thing called AIDS which no one could explain fully. They just knew it was bad. Where did it come from? How long has it been around? These were the questions being asked. No one knew the answers then and until the late 90s still did not know all the answers. I noticed a few coworkers who were on disability for only a short time at a company I worked for in 1984. Shortly after I had heard this the company informed us of their deaths. One died of pneumonia, and the other died of Kaposi's Sarcoma which to my knowledge only older men die from. We all knew it might be connected to this AIDS thing, but no one would discuss it.

Many people were afraid to talk about the virus. At times, it became dangerous to speak about it in public for fear that others would think the person discussing it had the virus. Guilt by verbal association. It sounded a bit medieval to me. But I wanted to learn more about it, so I decided to go to the library.

The New York Public Library is an impressive structure on 5th Ave. the side of Manhattan. Two huge resting lions flank the white marble stairs that lead up to the huge doors. I figured that a place so big and prestigious would have the answer or at least something to read about AIDS or caring for someone with it.

As I walked through the massive doors into the main lobby, I felt a little humbled by its sheer size. I walked up to the information desk and asked where I should go to find information on HIV/AIDS. The woman behind the desk directed me to another area where I met a librarian. I asked again, and the librarian told me they had nothing on the subject in book form but might have some articles. Imagine, a subject that could wipe out humanity hadn't made the bestseller list or the New York Library. Something was wrong with that, I thought.

The librarian noticed I was puzzled and asked me a few questions. He realized that I was looking for the caregiving aspect of AIDS as I knew a few people who were HIV positive. He said he only had technical nursing books on the shelves. As we spoke, he began to have a strange look on his face. He said to me "You might think I am crazy, but I do have a book, that if you were able to creatively translate the wording to apply to care for someone who may have a hard time communicating, it might be what you were looking for." The book was called Caring for Your Pet. Curious, I thought about it and eventually took his advice. Believe it or not, it worked in some instances as when Mark, for example, could not always tell me what he wanted or needed at the very end of his illness, so I had to anticipate it for a while. I watched eye movement and gestures and expressions that might give me a clue. When you are taking care of a pet, you must watch its expressions and gestures to understand what it might want or need. To this day I use this while working with kids who have a hard time expressing themselves.

Seeing that the subject of AIDS was not widely published, I began to think it was not too serious a disease. I wasn't sure what to do or where to go, so I went home. While I was on the train, I met someone who, in general, looked healthy, well dressed and appeared to have the world at his feet. We exchanged hellos and spoke about the weather. He mentioned how dreary the day was getting. That confused me as the days were sunny and warm with the promise of spring in the air. He asked me what I did and if I was from around here, as I did not have a standard New York accent. I told him about my past work as a store window designer, hoping he might have connections in the field and my photography which I was just getting interested in and that I had just moved here from New Hampshire a few years ago.

"Do you like New York?" he asked.

"I think so," I said. "I haven't spent too much time in the city. I was just in from the library today looking for some information about AIDS."

His presence became quieter, and he spoke less and less, but as usual, I babbled on. As I was talking about how hard it was to find my information about AIDS, he handed me a paper. It had the letters AIDS on it like the can I had questioned the bartender about earlier.

"What is this?" I asked.

"Here, take this and here is my number if you need more information," he said.

I asked, "Where did you get this?"

"My doctor," he said. "I have AIDS."

"Really?" I asked as if I were impressed. I didn't know what to say.

I wanted to ask him all kinds of questions, but I thought that it would be rude. The silence that followed was uncomfortable but lasted for the rest of the ride home.

When I got home, I read the material. I was shocked to read what this AIDS thing was and no one was saying or doing anything about it, as it seemed. My sympathy for this guy was overwhelming, and I felt powerless. I thought, do people know what this AIDS thing is all about? If they do why aren't they talking about it? Is there anything being done about it? Unfortunately, it was also called the Gay Disease which linked it to the prejudice society imposes on the gay community.

I thought about it a lot and finally got up enough nerve to call him to thank him for the information and also for being so courageous to be so open with me. I said, "I feel so sorry for you." His reply was, "Don't feel sorry. I am impressed. Most people won't even talk about it or speak to someone with it. I am glad you called and thank you for your concern. If I ever need to talk to someone, I will call you."

I felt good after I hung up. I felt like I had done some great service to humanity or something. Now I see it more clearly. What I had done was give that person a chance to share what was going on with him when no one else would listen.

That became an important day for me. It would also help me later on, with my caring for Mark. I would be able to listen to Mark and give him a line of communication most people with AIDS don't have access to. I never shared that with Mark but it was always there in the back of my mind.

When caring for anyone, I found that if you listen more than talk, the job or situation becomes a little more tolerable. I found it to be harder to listen totally to someone than talk, but when I did, it helped me do a better job as a Caregiver. To this day, working with kids in school and listening to them makes all the difference. We as teachers, Caregivers or educated ones, many times, dismiss the fact that they have a lot to say. My experiences as an outspoken teenager and seeing those kids in Florida speak up about the school shootings are proof that they can make a difference. I also found it is as important in the learning process while teaching them. To give them a voice or a chance to vent opens a whole new avenue to the learning process and increases the level of self-esteem and trust between teacher/aide and student.

I am finding as I get older, all the time I spent as a Caregiver and student of life has given me an edge while working with the kids I work with now. Many of them are kids who have no tolerance for being in the classroom for many reasons. Others use violence and abusive language to compensate for their being so uncomfortable. Being able to listen and then assess the true situation and the reasons why they are acting out makes such a difference in the quality of their school experience. In most cases in the school system, the supervisors and Special Ed Coordinators are the ones who know the whole story. The person who is working directly with the student, in many cases, has limited access to the whole story, and because they are working directly with the student, they should know much more than they do. I know that is not true for some schools, but it was my experience in some of the situations I was working in.

Many times, because it is so disturbing and disruptive, they are just sent home to where the problem might have originated. Once a student is stabilized, we can get on with the work of assisting them in their school work allowing them to teach us how to teach them. Each child is an individual and has their own history. Knowing this and using this to the teacher's advantage allows us to decompress them, if you will, and give them a chance to learn. The key is to find out what their passion is. Knowing what that passion is can be vital as a tool in teaching. Many times, I have gone back to that passion for bringing them back into the learning process. It becomes familiar again, and they become open to conversation and more. When I say passion, it could be their interest in cars, sports or something they have a strong interest in.

My own experience with this as a straight D student in high school was when the teachers could not understand why I was failing. I would answer just six questions usually and turn it in. My guidance counselor called me to his office and at a time when Attention Deficit Disorder was not a known thing, I realized that after six questions I would lose concentration and get fidgety. I began to take my tests in his office, and after I could not go any further on the test he would say, "Let's take a walk or go play basketball." This would divert the ADD situation, and when I came back, I was able to finish the test. My grades went up, and I had a good dose of self-esteem which I did not have before. He would also discuss my passion, which changed weekly.

Working as a Para Educator, now known as Educational Technician, and a one-on-one Personal Care Attendant or PCA has led me to understand that even in that role I am a Caregiver. It also allows me to use my experience to the fullest. There are many ways to teach but to have that base where the student can feel comfortable enough to learn by you listening more, to me, is the key to success. I feel you can't teach, help or successfully change the social environment around you unless you first listen, and I mean really listen with no preaching, talking or advising of any sort. Then when the listening has been exhausted, the teaching and the change begins. This is something I think the government or Congress could do a little more of.

ELSIE'S GARDEN

The day I moved to College Point, New York, a section of Queens, was an unsettling day for me.

There was a sense of fear, uncertainty, excitement and newness I hadn't felt since I had gone to Brazil in 1971. When I went to Brazil, I knew I would return a year later to the warmth, comfort, familiarities, and security of my family. This time I wasn't going home in that sense, in fact, I wasn't sure what was going to happen at all. No job, no security and no idea what was ahead of me. This was a real shot in the dark. The apartment I would be moving into was on the opposite side of the road from a waterfront property which was on the Flushing Bay. If you stood at the water's edge, or at my living room window, you could see LaGuardia Airport. It was indeed not the quietest location, but after a while, I got used to it.

Across the street from my apartment stood a house that seemed to have been the result of time standing still. It needed work, and God knows it must have weathered some heavy storms in its lifetime. It stood high enough though from the water to keep the bay water out. Although I am sure a hefty Nor'easter could have dampened its spirits.

On the left side of the house as you face it was an overgrown garden full of a variety of common and unusual plants, roses, fig trees, apple trees, Black-Eyed Susan, a grapevine which needed help and some boxwood bushes planted by the owner from cuttings many years prior. These bushes were now bubbling out in their molten shape as if they refused to conform to the hedge clippers' idea of sculpture. The weeds seemed to be the most common plants. It was kind of an oasis in an area that had been taken over by new construction and a lot of old buildings that were remodeled each with a facelift that would keep up with the times.

Behind the green-shuttered, wide clapboard house with its 12 over 12 paned windows overlooking the bay was the grape yard and a collection of garden implements rusting in the open air and in some cases oxidized beyond recognition. There was evidence of some attempt to save them, as they were covered with a few pieces of plastic as if someone in a rush had tried to protect them from the elements. Many of the wooden items had black charcoal on them as if they had been in a fire at some point. In the middle of the yard, there were a series of cotton rope lines with fragments of cloth rags on them blowing in the breeze. The lines led up to the garage and a cabana, long past its glory days and in need of a paint job.

After getting settled in my apartment I had just acquired, which was directly across the street from this relic of a house, I would sit in my front window and look out over the bay. I would admire the house and garden with the white picket fence in the foreground and a gleaming cityscape behind it wondering if those two worlds ever met. On warm days, I would see the couple who lived there, sitting out on the north side of the house where there was a little makeshift patio under the chestnut tree surrounded by a rainbow of colored flowers. Against the house was a bench that seemed like it might have come out of a church or school at one time. It was well weathered and had seen better days. The old guy who was usually seen with a walker would sit on the bench and be attended by a short white-haired teddy bear of a woman who was always on the go and getting things for him. They were in their 80s and looked like they had owned the house for a long time.

Most of my days were spent looking for a job in the city. Not knowing much about New York City, it was a slow process. Coming home to the apartment, I would walk down a side street that ended with an oasis-like setting with the house diagonally on the left across the street and a dead-end that leads to the back of their house and the bay.

Coming back home from my daily search for a job, I encountered the couple sitting outside, she with a cup of tea and he with a beer-filled glass, and the can close by. I waved, trying to be polite and a good neighbor and they waved back. Feeling the need to connect I decided to go over to them and introduce myself. They were the first friendly people I have met in my new neighborhood, not that I ventured out much for fear of getting lost, but most people I encountered were seemingly on a mission or just in one damn hurry. I walked up to the gate which was painted an old cracked white finish which, I am sure in its lifetime has allowed a myriad of characters through the wooden fortress that led to this shaded garden and the front steps of the house. The gate was in desperate need of paint but seeing their age, I understood the condition of the house. It was like everything behind the gate had been frozen in time. It was an unusual sight in an area that was dealing with the encroachment of society and industry.

The woman, short, a little bow-legged with a stained apron introduced herself as Elsie and then said, "This is my husband, Frank." I waved to him, but he just raised his hand clutching his beer and grunted. It was obvious he was at a difficult time in his life, not being able to do many of the things he had loved to do in his younger years. I noticed that he had a walker next to him which indicated that his life may have been rudely interrupted by illness and explained his periodic grunts of disgust. Elsie invited me over to the cement block patio to sit with them a spell and chat with them, so I did. Frank was a matter of fact kind of guy. I could see he must have had an interesting life. I listened to what became a long line of stories ranging from how to make sauerkraut and applejack to his work as an engineer in the local factories.

These were proud people and very resourceful. They saved everything, not unlike what my dad did. This act of saving things was an activity well documented and stemmed from the depression when even the smallest string was something of value. If something has even the remotest possibility of being used again, they were willing to give it another life. This included paper and plastic bags, wood, cloth, and containers. Yet even with all this clutter it was organized and seemed to always have an appropriate place. I look at how I have been altering my life in these hard times as a Caregiver and still working two jobs. I still recycle as much as possible and save anything I think I might be able to use in the future, something I am working on changing daily.

Frank's condition stemmed from when he had fallen and broken both hips. This left him with a walker, and it wasn't getting any better. Seeing they could use some help I told them that if they ever needed a hand with something to please call me and I would come over. Another instance when the Caregiver side of me popped up. It wasn't long before I was called over to help Frank go up the stairs as Elsie was getting scared that he might fall and hurt himself again. She was also pretty unstable herself with her footing not being what it used to be. With her age and being so frail, it was a wonder she hadn't fallen with him and both gotten hurt already. I didn't know it then but everything I would be experiencing with them over the next several years would be a training ground for my stamina and patience as a Caregiver.

Over the next few years, I would learn many things from Frank. He had story after story to tell, and they were all true. Sometimes he would tell me a story and I would have doubts about it and would say, "Really?" His response would be, "I don't bullshit anyone." He also told me, "Whenever you dish out the bullshit you always end up with the shovel to clean it up somewhere down the road."

He was full of these anecdotes and philosophies. I, at age 34, was eager to listen. Here was a man who had seen two world wars, grew up with only a mother to raise him and worked his way through many hard times including the depression. He was always willing to share it with anyone who would listen to him.

While we spoke, sometimes over a beer, Elsie would come in to listen. Frank immediately stopped talking and would give out a huff and wave her off saying, "89 years in this house gives me the right to tell my stories without any interruption." He had seen the street he lived on and the town he lived in change over the years. He was around when the pictures in the Poppenhusen Institute, one of the first educationally oriented public programs of its type founded by Mr. Poppenhusen and funded in part by his friend Andrew Carnage, were taken of the town and surrounding areas in the late 1890s. Elsie used to take classes at the Institute when she was a little girl. It also housed the first public kindergarten in the United States.

College Point had been a secluded area with only a few ways to get into it. It was much like a resort area with boathouses and swimming areas all around. For many years it was untouched by the progress around it. As Queens and New York City grew, it stayed the same for the most part. Around 1930 it was discovered by developers and the physical makeup of the community began to grow. Many of the changes came about when the 1939 New York World's Fair became a focal point of the area and altered the culture dramatically. I realized that Frank was a wealth of information about this area of New York.

As time passed, simple tasks became more difficult for Frank as it became harder and harder for Elsie to help him. His stair climbing days were over, and they had to bring in a hospital bed putting it in the living room on the first floor where Elsie would have no problem working with him. It was also easier for the nurse to help him as the kitchen, as small and compact as it was, was just a room away. The living room became his world and the window next to his chair where he sat all day, became his only access to the outside world which was now going on, business as usual, without him.

Over the next few years, we became very close friends. It was rare for me to come straight home without going over to check on them. I did errands for them and helped them with house repairs normally supervised by Frank. He was the eyes and the brain, and I was his hands and legs. I always felt it must have been rough for him having been the handyman and at times inventor, to have to sit on the sidelines.

One night Elsie called me and asked me to help Frank as he had to go to the bathroom. It was 3:00 A.M., and I had to get up in a couple of hours to go to work. I went over and lifted him out of bed and put him on the portable toilet the nurse had brought in for him. There we sat and discussed the world events.

About 30 minutes later he looked at me and said, "Don't be mad at me but it was a false alarm." He apologized again, and I carried him back to the bed. Luckily, he was only about 80 lbs. When he was settled, I asked Elsie if there was anything she needed. She said, "I don't think so." She thanked me again and again as I walked out the door. Walking across the street to my apartment I noticed her figure in the window waving to me.

Just a few months earlier, Chuck, had gotten married and there was a room in the apartment open. I had just met Mark at a club in Queens. We had become great friends. He was into design, graphics, and photography as was I. We liked biking and the beach. I had finally met someone in New York who was compatible, and we enjoyed each other's company. He moved in shortly after we met as I needed a roommate to share the expenses and he had to move out of his apartment house for renovations. I think the building was going co-op, but we did not find out until much later. Good old New York free enterprise. The apartment he lived in, which was only two rooms, cost him about $450 a month and was now going for $1200 a month.

When I got home from helping Frank, Mark was in the kitchen with a glass of water in his hand. He couldn't understand what I was doing out at 3:30 A.M. in my bathrobe. I told him about Frank. He shook his head from side to side with a sleepy acknowledgment, "Doing a great job." Then I went to bed. Mark never questioned my doing this. He felt it was just who I was. He seldom mentioned it until after he was ill for some time. We were sitting in the hospital where he had just undergone radiation therapy. He mentioned that he had not said anything about my caring for Frank and Elsie and had to admit it bothered him sometimes. At the time, he felt I was giving up a lot of my own time for them. Then he said, "Now I understand why you did it and who you are. You are a real Caregiver." He paused with his head down and his eyes looking up at me saying, "Thanks." He then proceeded to vomit from the treatment.

Back to Elsie. In the weeks and months to come, I would be called over almost once a night to help Frank. At first, it was difficult, but it later became just something I did. I think a lot of the reason I didn't mind helping was that I learned so much from Frank, not so much from what he spoke about but to get a glimpse of what it was like to grow old and how much we rely on each other at any age. What I didn't know then was that in just a few years I would be helping Mark.

One day after coming home from the city, I saw an ambulance in front of Frank and Elsie's house. When I investigated a little more and walked over to the paramedics, they were carrying Frank into the ambulance. It seemed he was smoking and his shirt caught fire. Even though he didn't have all his senses up and running, the expression on his face was one that said, "Oh well, chalk up another one for me." He almost had an intoxicating look about him. But he was off for another ride. It was almost like this was the only way he could get some excitement in his life. Not that he did it on purpose, but when things like this happened, he seemed to enjoy the experience with vigor. Elsie put her arm around me as her body shook from sobbing. I told her that this was a blessing in disguise, that she could get some rest and have some time to herself. She agreed and went into the house, asking me to sit with her and have a cup of tea. I accepted.

Seeing how Elsie was able to go through this and how she had the strength to endure it, to this day amazes me. Going through Mark's illness at my age was hard enough but Elsie at 85, I could only imagine the toll it took on her. Some of the strength I had came from helping her with Frank and watching how she cared for him and it gave me the incentive to be with Mark to the end. I used to see her go into a mode of being on automatic. She was doing what she thought she had to do.

When Frank died, which was not too long after the cigarette incident, Elsie was with him. She told me how he stopped breathing, the gasp for breath and the eventual gurgle with not much emotion but just as a matter of fact as a nurse or doctor would. She spent almost 70 years with Frank and now he was gone. "It was so peaceful when he left. He was out of his misery and in a quiet place" she said softly.

Her strength during the funeral and all the events that followed gave me strength that I would carry with me through to Mark's graveside. It was then, at the funeral, I felt we all needed to lean on each other.

The few years to follow were filled with laughs and trip like trips to the city, attending the opera and community events. We shared many hours together, and this was my first experience in making each moment count even if I didn't want to right then. She taught me that when you get older, you find out how short life is, and that if you do not make the best of each moment you can regret not having done things. Elsie was a person who lived life simply but with fullness and purpose. This time with her was a special time in my life, and its teachings would carry me through my dad's death and Mark's. I remember we had a birthday party for her. She had more energy than most of us who were younger. Her godson made a comment that "knowing Elsie she'll be here long after we go." It was like we didn't want her to go, as we would feed off her energy and zest for life.

As the weeks went on after the party, I noticed she was not doing well. I could see that all the events in recent times while caregiving was taking a toll on her even though we all thought she would live forever. A day without Elsie? Absurd. One evening she was beginning to see things that weren't there. When I arrived, she was being taken to the hospital. I followed the ambulance with her niece. She was one of Elsie's closest relatives.

When we arrived at the hospital, we were told they would have to admit her for observation. I decided to go home. When I got back to my apartment, I told Mark what had happened. I could see it affected him yet he would not show it. However, he did say to me, "If there is anything I can do, let me know." I knew he didn't want to be a part of it as he felt uncomfortable with things like this, but just to hear him offer help was enough to let me know he cared and understood what I was going through. It's amazing how that little sign of support can go a long way to save one's sanity.

While she was in the hospital, I went to see her several times. The last time I was there I sat in her room next to her bed. Here, this woman with so much energy and love was curled up, catheterized and in pain. I reached through the bed guard, which looked like bars from prison, to hold her hand. She looked like a baby, scared and frail. The nurse had told me not to be upset if she didn't recognize me. She hadn't been able to recognize many people and hadn't responded too well to physical touch. It was apparent she had just had a stroke.

I held her hand for a moment and spoke to her about all the things that had been going on outside the hospital. I told her about the weather and how Mark was doing. As I spoke, she began to pull my hand closer to her and had a tight hold on my fingers. As she pulled my arm over to her, she pulled herself closer to the railing and held it with the other hand. Her mouth was not functioning well because of the stroke. It looked like she had just come from the dentist and her face was still numb.

As she looked at me, my eyes were wet with tears. She began to mumble. What I heard after the third try was, "we had a great friendship, didn't we?" Well, I lost it right about then. I just sat there not knowing what to say. After pulling myself together a bit, I replied, "Yes, we did Elsie, we surely did."

I waited for her sister to come in and sit with her. I didn't want to leave as she held on for dear life and I knew she didn't want me to go. When her sister came in she had some other people with her which bothered me and might have been why Elsie was so unresponsive to her sister. I know I would not have felt comfortable with a group of people hovering over me if I was in her state. However, I thought she needed time with her family, and I quietly whispered to her to let her know I would be back the next day. As I left, I whispered to her that I loved her. She looked at me with a big old tear landing on her pillow.

I leaned over and kissed her on the cheek. I knew she wanted it to end so she could be with Frank. As I left and walked down the hall, I thought of all the lessons she had taught me, especially about how important it was to be strong yet caring. I found that relationships like this one were few and far between. Many times they only happen if we let them. I have tried to use this philosophy in my caregiving episodes. Memories were whizzing through my head like bullets.

When I got home, I told Mark what happened. He felt sad for me that I had just spent so much time helping Frank and Elsie and it had come to this. We talked about it for a while. Mark, not being one to belabor things said, almost interrupting himself, "Let's go out to eat. You need to get away." We did, and I was fine.

Elsie had influenced our lives like no one else. Mark always referred to her backyard full of debris as Elsie's Garden. Most of it was junk that she had kept there for Frank to fix when he got better. Frank never got better, yet she did this with many of his things in the basement and around the house, sometimes even after his death. Things in his bedroom were just as they were when he became ill. I found myself doing the same thing as with Mark and my friend Burt who you will meet later in the book.

I would buy things that we could use later when he got better, Mark never got better. I found myself doing the same, even after his death. It was like I had to hold onto things the way they were just in case it was all a dream or something. Years later, I wanted to build a chapel attached to the house in VT and collected church things like altars, windows and crosses, and even an organ. Burt never got better either. I also found after talking to many people who have lost loved ones that this is very normal and it shouldn't be questioned by others. It is all a part of the healing process. My garden with all its chaos was a little more organized and less cluttered than Elsie's, but the concept was still the same.

A couple of days after that emotional meeting in the hospital, Elsie died. The memories I have of her as a ball of energy and kindness will always stay with me. After the funeral, I took some time to go to her garden and remind myself of what I had just experienced as Elsies Caregiver. Her clothesline, still with rags drying in the wind, the grapevine with the unpicked shriveled grapes still there from the fall and harsh winter hang motionless in the light breeze as a testimonial that she did exist once. To the side were old pots that never got new plants because she was taking care of Frank. A shovel, that still stands leaning against the house rusted to the point of extinction leaves its age mark on the white-painted house. Then there was the anvil where Frank made many of the creations that made Elsie's life a little easier was pressed against the cement by its weight. The old cactus bed we didn't get to cover with plastic last year to protect it from the cold which didn't make it for the first time since she had planted them in the 50s lay rotted ready to fertilize the soil. All of the things which were part of her and Frank's existence were now disappearing. She wasn't here anymore to care for her garden, and unless someone could tend to it, it would surely disappear.

Mark had always wanted to do a photo essay called Elsie's Garden. I had hoped he would, but it never happened. Without Elsie to take care of, I felt lost and yet free to continue my life. These were difficult opposing feelings to deal with. The good thing was that I felt complete with her and Frank. I don't feel there was much unsaid.

Several years later Mark died. I returned to her house in Queens only to find an unkempt garden full of weeds and trees. Most of the debris was gone, and the windows boarded up. The house was up for sale. It was the end of an era for this little old house. Soon it would either be gone or have another life. I prayed for the latter.

Before Elsie died, the house next door had been sold. Elsie had a soft spot in her heart for it. The company across the street had bought it and had plans to make office space in its place.

One morning I woke up to a noise that startled me. I looked out the window, and there was Elsie on the corner, sitting in a folding chair preparing to watch the demolition of her neighbor's house. As a photographer, I thought it would be a good opportunity for some fantastic shots. I didn't know how right I was. The collapse of the building has become a permanent part of an exhibit of mine called,

"Faded Dreams Broken Windows" which is a collection of old pieces of buildings, articles, tires, and gardens which were once someone's dream and now only hold memories which can only be reclaimed through stories and broken windows. I knew what Elsie was feeling that day the house fell.

I realized, after my walk through the quiet unkempt garden, that we move in cycles. We live, we learn, we grow, and then we grow old and die. Sometimes we don't get to grow old. We just die. I was comfortable with that. I believe this knowledge made me strong enough to go through the losses I have gone through. Elsie became my strength and one of my teachers in life. I often wonder why we go through the things we do and where it will all bring us to. We spend all our lives growing, loving and creating only to end up in a beautifully built, padded casket or a box full of ashes. There must be something more.

Turning back to the church after so many years has given me hope and calmness that carries me through the days. Even if I have doubts and questions about religion and God, I feel it is something to hold on to and can give me some peace.

I believe, therefore, that Mom, Dad, Frank, Elsie, Mark, and Burt are still with me. I only wish I could have felt this way with them while they were alive. This is why I cherish all of my relationships and encounters with people I am with today even the ones I wished I had not met. We are here but a short time. To waste the knowledge I have received from these loving, caring people, would be sad.

We all lose something through death, but if we allow it, we can acknowledge the gains we make through these losses and create fuller and better lives while we are here. I used to be afraid of death. Now I accept it as part of life and the greater story yet to be told.

The Calm Before the Storm

After Elsie's death, Mark had gained employment in Stamford Ct., at Tommy Hilfiger. He became a manager and worked many hours. I was still working freelance in New York City. However, I was spending over an hour to get to work and yet could see the building I worked in from my living room. Only in New York.

There had been recent problems and threats from the tenant below us. Mark's tax return had not arrived yet so he called to find out when it would arrive. He was surprised to hear that it had been sent and was cashed already so he requested a copy of the endorsement and where it was cashed.

When the letter arrived several weeks later, he found out that the mother of the tenant below us who had caused him so much trouble had co-signed it with the signature of the tenant and deposited it into her account. Mark quickly confronted the guy only to get thrown through the door. He came upstairs and said, "I am leaving and if you want to stay you can, but I am history." He packed and took off for his mothers' house in New Jersey.

For a month, he stayed at his mothers' house. During this time, he made plans to move to Stamford Connecticut. I got a call from him inviting me to look at an apartment there. I was not planning on moving, so it would be difficult to go with him, but with all that had happened, it began to look like a good idea.

When I saw the apartment, I couldn't say no. It was big, not far from a train station where the trip only took 30 minutes with the express train compared to an hour from Queens. The cost was less than my old apartment, and we each had a bedroom and an office we could share. To say no now would stress our friendship and lessen the trust. I had to say yes.

Papers were signed, and within a couple of months, I could move in and begin a new life in Connecticut. Leaving Queens, I felt I was leaving a part of a journey I had found myself on. I hoped that it was the end of me being a Caregiver. Soon I would find out how far from the end I was.

Life was a little different in the suburbs which lowered my stress. We could walk down the street, and it was a real neighborhood, much like where I grew up. I began to go to church and met many people who would become some of my closest friends. Yet I was also close to New York City which I loved dearly. Life became good. I could explore my photography talent and was accepted as a board member of the Stamford Arts Society. It was a position I could continue networking with and expand my photography interests. Most of the people who were on the board were well-to-do, and I felt out of place at times, but I was able to adjust to the differences and my low self-esteem.

Two years had passed since the big move. Mark began to show signs of having a serious problem health-wise, and I was soon to find out he was HIV Positive. My job as a Caregiver was officially reinstated now. For several months, I noticed that Mark was getting weaker and weaker. Until now his diagnosis was "just a diagnosis." It became real. He intended to fight this thing to the end. This was when being diagnosed was pretty much a death sentence. For about 16 months he would go to the Gym every day. Being concerned about his welfare I went with him and began to feel that he might beat this after all. He was healthy and eating well. His attitude was great, and the doctor was pleased with his progress and attitude. His hard work was paying off. Things were beginning to look good. At the time, we both thought we would be in this place in time, called wellness, at least for a while. Anyone I knew who got the diagnosis had gotten sick and sort of disappeared. It seemed, or at least I had hoped, that this was not the case with Mark.

Our energy was positive, no pun intended, and we had made many plans. We were going to travel and experience life to the fullest. This was a good time to do the many things we wanted to do now that we both had this kick in the pants and a new awareness about life and how short it could be. It seemed nothing could stop us now. We were invulnerable as a team. It was like I felt when I was a teenager. Our friendship had grown stronger than ever. My goal was to make sure he was going to be ok, and his goal was to get better and stay healthy.

A friend of mine asked me how we could have such a strong friendship for so long. His question took me back a bit, but I thought about it. It is trust and commitment and honesty that made our friendship so strong. I have taken that theory to each of my friendships. If there is little trust or the trust is broken, the friendship has little foundation to grow on.

Sure, little things would slow him down, but they were only small potholes in the road. People were giving him hope. This made me stronger as well. The media and news programs that were geared to the AIDS pandemic had all kinds of promise by now for a cure. Nothing concrete, but a lot of promise. We both lived in hope. Even the doctor would say that he was doing well and to keep up with the good eating and exercise.

It was the calm before the storm, now that I think about it. We were enjoying life and all it had to offer. He sometimes said, "I want to live like I am dying". Christmas came and went. We began to plan trips and things we were going to do in the future. He was going to live forever. When I think back to that time, I can relive the feelings of wonderful expectations and yet there was always that occasional dark cloud that would remind me that "we" were still fighting for his life.

There was one day when the sun came out after a series of rainy days. He had been feeling weaker and weaker but still working 60 hours and trying to enjoy life and beat the odds. But this day with the sun out he wasn't feeling his best yet, we both wanted to take advantage of the moment. He suggested that we take a drive to a wooded area close to where we lived. Wooded areas were few and far between in Stamford, and we both enjoyed hiking and climbing. It was all he could do to get ready to go, but the sun was out, and it was time. We just had to go. He was showing signs of tiring, but the fight in him was still strong. It is funny how now I see how sick he was, but when you are that close for so long, the changes are slow and hard to notice in the moment. We got to the wooded area and began to walk. I noticed he was looking around for something, picking up branches and throwing them aside. He finally found a stick that became his walking stick and then we were off to enjoy the moment. I could see his pain but said nothing. I believe he actually was enjoying the woods and the occasional animal or bird that passed by despite the pain which was obvious.

We got to a brook where we sat and talked for a while. He mostly spoke of how good it was to smell the clean, fresh air. We threw a few rocks in the water and sat quietly.

Suddenly I could see the panic in his face. He quickly said, "let's go, it is getting too much for me."

When I said, "are you sure you don't want to just sit a while longer?" he yelled, "no! I want to go now."

As we began to walk back to the car, I had my camera with me as usual and began to take pictures. While taking pictures, I didn't have to think. This got him more upset and he said, "Put that damn thing away and let's go back." The same camera he gave me for Christmas in hopes of me becoming a great photographer was now a target of his pain. I let him go ahead of me while I snuck a few more shots. One of the shots I got was of him up ahead leaning on his walking stick as he grumbled walking at the end of the dirt road.

I didn't know what that picture would mean to me later, but when I look at it now, I see the beginning of the storm surge. It is embedded in my mind as the end of the calm.

When we got back home, he got to the top of the stairs and sat. "Get the key," he said, "I can't." I fumbled around looking for my key knowing he was in pain. "Hurry!" he yelled. I got the door open, and he went into the living room, took the pillow off the couch and pulled the afghan over him on the floor. It was an event that would become commonplace in days and weeks to come. When I asked him if I could get him something? He said in a shaky voice, "No! Just leave me alone."

I sat for a long time, quiet and scared. I don't know how long it was, but it seemed like forever. I didn't know what to do or say or what was going to happen. It is a tough place to be for a Caregiver. I began to think about how quickly things can change in situations like this. Going from such a good place with hopes and dreams to a place of fear and uncertainty was something I thought I understood until now. It was personal and would be something I would be very aware of in my future caregiving experiences.

From that point on, things got intense. Turmoil was standing on our doorstep. I felt I was slowly losing a friend to a monster killer. As if it were a storm, I began to prepare myself. I was not sure what I was preparing for; I just did things that seemed as if they needed to be done. I even made chicken soup from scratch, (yes from scratch). When I was a kid and times got tough, Mom always seemed to come up with soup of some kind. Funny how we become our parents.

In the days to follow, there was a lot of anger. I was as scared as he was. It was time to put my life on hold and begin caring for him but I didn't know how I was supposed to do that. There were no books or instruction manuals on how I was supposed to be a Caregiver. I just did it. For a while, he would just go to work and come home, put a pillow on the floor and cover himself with the afghan. I felt so alone and helpless somehow.

The old Mark took a leave of absence. A new Mark emerged. His fever was constant. His anger was increasing. His doctor helped me through a lot of it, but it never seemed to be enough. I thank God that his doctor did not have the usual requirements of being a relative or partner to get instructions and information on how to help. To him, we were partners in this stage of life. These days I see people still helpless because the hospitals will not let anyone but their relatives in on the deal. My biggest fear was that Mark was going to give up. With literally no one else I could feel comfortable talking to I began to talk to my minister. His words were like a breath of fresh air, but only for a moment. The storm was still raging, and I was still paddling upstream against the current. However, I wasn't going to give up.

One morning I got up and went into the kitchen only to find Mark making breakfast. To say the least, I was ready to cry. Taking the opportunity to the fullest, I sat a while talking to him. His spirit was back, and fever is gone. Mark was back, but for how long?

There were several episodes like that one in the following months. We came to realize that we needed each other to work together and fight this thing head-on. We must have only spoken for an hour, but it seemed like much more than one. It was just good to see him back. We knew it wasn't the end of his pain. It was only the eye of the storm. We decided to try and recognize when those calmer moments appeared and to take full advantage of them. That would be hard as we both had different careers and commitments. I had to be the flexible one no matter what mood I was in. As Caregiver, I quickly learned that I was in his world and was the one who had to adjust. Just knowing we were going to try to make it all work was enough to keep us going.

In most of my Caregiver jobs, I look back at this time as my education. I was learning by the seat of my pants, but it would prove to be well worth it. Anyone who is a Caregiver can most likely relate to this chapter. Not becoming angry and abusive is hard as it is a natural defense. Nurses are trained to be aware of these things and can tell you how difficult it can be. In the hospital, the patient is usually not a loved one so there is a natural separation in place, plus it can become routine. With loved ones, it is so hard as the closeness can be the enemy.

My suggestion to anyone who is taking care of family, friend or someone this close, is to talk to nurses and other professionals and seek help emotionally. Many times, the Caregiver, in this case, can be the sicker one. By sicker, I mean emotionally and physically as it can be tiring.

Go with the flow and when you see the calm or the eye of the storm, take full advantage of it and know it is usually not very long. Be strong but be wise. Take care of yourself also.

THE GARDEN GATE

During the time Mark was still well enough to work, walk and lead a relatively normal life, he found it important to plan things that would make life more functional, calm and in general, livable.

One of those times was in January 1992. It had been a rough winter, and he needed to get away.

Quite frankly I felt then and still feel today that I needed to get away more, as I was working in New York City, taking a couple of photography courses and taking care of Mark on my downtime. I never whined about it to him, as that would have made it a competition as to who needed it more and I didn't want to get into that. I found out later how no matter who it is giving care when someone is sick, the sickness will dominate the world of that person and drag everyone around them into that world like a black hole. This is especially true for terminal illnesses.

We had taken a few short trips and done some activities in the city, but it was not enough. He seemed to realize that there was little time left to do the things he needed to do which explained why we were both involved in this black hole. He felt that being HIV positive was pretty much a death sentence and was very free to express that.

He had asked me what week I thought would be a good week to go somewhere. My schedule, being more flexible, I decided to leave it up to him. I could plan around it as I was working freelance jobs at this point. He had heard that Cancun was a place that was worth going to and he had never been out of the country. He had always envied me for having gone to Brazil for more than a year and all the other countries I had visited. When I went to Poland, he got a kick out of talking to me on the phone. The idea of taking a week off became more and more enticing as we spoke about it.

Mark had asked a coworker and a great friend to stay at the apartment and watch the cat, Tugger, named after the character Rum Tum Tugger in the Broadway musical Cats, for his personality. If Tugger was in, he wasn't sure if he should stay in or go out, and when he got out he wasn't sure if he should go in or stay out. He also thought he was better and more handsome than most cats. Mark's friend agreed to stay, which took a load off our minds.

Suddenly we were off to experience and share what was to become one of the most beautiful and spiritual vacations either of us had taken. Even better than Disney World, which for me was hard to beat. You see, I had worn the costume of Winnie the Pooh for Sears and traveled with it for a while. Winnie or Pooh is still one of my nicknames. I had to go to Disney World unofficially to train in the costume. It was sweaty and hot, but I loved every minute of it. To go to the place where Winnie was developed as a star character and meet him there was like meeting my idol. It was the highpoint of my life until Cancun. Cancun was one we both made special given the circumstances. I knew it might be the last trip he would be taking, so I wanted it to be special.

While we were in the lobby of the hotel, we met two guys from the Philippines who were staying there. We had been planning some side trips, as were they. Mark, having a zest for learning about and meeting new cultures, thought it would be a great opportunity to get to know them and make some of the side trips together. I had already introduced myself when Mark came over. When we asked them what country they were from, they said they were from New York. Talk about culture shock! We have since become great friends. They both became Mark's new special people. They were willing to share their trip with us. Through meeting them, Mark began to open up to others about his being HIV positive. They were more open to listening than most people he had met. He began to see the beautiful side of society with all its cultural differences, and they were totally accepting of Mark.

During the week, he made a comment that he thought he would like to attend church or at least go in one. This was new to me to see him interested in church. It seemed like he wanted to do as much as possible, and church seemed to fit the bill. We took a cab to get into the old town of Cancun which was less glitzy and very poor. While we were in the cab, I spoke to the driver in broken Spanish or modified Portuguese which I speak fluently. Mark was so impressed I could speak another language. I was just hoping he would not feel bad that he never learned another language. We got out of the cab and walked into a little chapel which was very Mexican in style. His silence and curiosity were especially interesting to me as I have never seen him so solemn. It was as if he became aware of his spirituality at that moment. He spent some time there very quiet, and I just let him. Then, as if he awoke from sleep, he got up and said "let's go".

Later that week the challenge of climbing up the Mayan pyramids, which represented a spiritual ideal of the past, became important to him. It also moved me despite the stories of the human sacrifices that took place there. The thrill he got from getting to the top helped him touch something that was untouchable before. His love for life was changing for the better. Later while in the hospital before his death, he said that he wished he had always lived his life like he has lived it the past few years. Even though the climb exhausted him, he felt he touched something spiritually significant.

We were lucky in that way that we could afford to do these things even on our tight budgets but it was a lesson I took well. I only wonder about the people who, because of HIV, lost their jobs, insurance, and life savings and can not do the things they needed to do to be complete. Then I think of the people we see on the street with their signs about having AIDS and a cup in their hand, begging for money or just the sandwich you may not have eaten at lunch. It was an awakening I will always remember and since then I have tried to make a difference by talking to people and sharing my experience. Although there are many times when they do not want to hear it they can pass judgment on me and put me in a box I cannot fit in. I try my best to get past that. Yet the number of times I have shared my experience with others that have made a positive difference outweighs the negative. Since then I have worked at The Sharing Community, which is a program dedicated to helping the homeless, substance abusers, the hungry and HIV/AIDS. It is there I have been able to make the biggest difference. I also work with kids in the school system, and even though I have been criticized for not having the degree to be able to help the more violent kids, they still send them my way and after 12 years, have not questioned my techniques or the stories I tell them.

I find the school system is so outdated in many ways and cannot deal with many of the social and emotional issues caused by family life, peer pressure, and drug availability. They are in competition with MTV, computer games, iPad and all those reality shows which do not bleep anything out and subliminally say it is ok to hit, fight, swear, smoke and do drugs. I wonder where this spiral and technological permissiveness will end.

An experience I had with Mark while taking him to the radiation clinic in New York, struck a tough note with me. I had just gotten him into the wheelchair and was wheeling him to the door when we passed one of the many homeless people on the street. In front of him was a sign which read, "I have AIDS. Don't be afraid. Please help me get a meal or give me some of your leftover lunch. I want to live." This sent shivers through my body as I wheeled Mark by him. I thought to myself that the last part of his sign should read "I want to exist".

I knew Mark saw him. We just wheeled by him because Mark didn't want to be late for his appointment. After we got into the doorway, he stopped me. He turned, looked at me and said, "If I ever yell at you or complain again, shut me up." The experience went deep, and I think it helped our quality time together. Being his Caregiver and friend, I wanted the best for him. I didn't want him sitting on the side of the road begging to exist.

One evening in Cancun one evening we were taking a walk after dinner at one of those tourist trap restaurants. The sun was just about to set. He never has shown much interest in sunsets before, but this one seemed important. We sat on a grassy bank near the water and watched the sun slowly set. Not a word was said. It was so symbolic then, and every time I get the chance to see a sunset, I think of that day in Cancun, Mexico.

The quietness and spiritual quality of that day were profound. It was almost as if we had found the garden gate and realized we had the key all along. I open it as often as I can now and have found it to be a garden full of wonder and love. The gate represents the opportunity to look at life positively and see all it can offer. Of course, there are the inevitable weeds and bugs, but as long as I can see the garden, I can tend to the weeds. It is the pain and uncertainties which overpower the garden that make the gardening or living difficult. Yet the garden is still there. It is a little like Elsie's garden.

I think Mark, his parents and I saw the garden clearer than ever with all of us weeding it together. It became wonderful even with the biggest and ugliest weed called AIDS. This type of support is something that I feel is needed with the experience of AIDS, diabetes, Alzheimer's, Dementia, caregiving and any other illness or situation that changes one's life so much that it makes us look at our mortality. A little smile or friendly word occasionally was all that was needed.

My friends in St John's Church in Stamford Ct, Nellie, Janet, Julie and Elizabeth, who have all passed away, were part of my garden at that time. They were in the rose section. Nellie's help with getting the wheelchair for Mark, Janet's wonderful soups and salads, Julie's friendly discussions around her dining room table and Elizabeth with her friendly hello and genuine concern for me became moments I can never begin to fully repay or express enough thanks for.

Of course, in the center of the garden was Mark. Like a fountain, his jokes, (practical or not), his laugh and his concern for those who were caring for him flowed right up to the last days in the hospital.

You may think that with all this garden stuff, I must be losing it. I don't think so. Everyone has a garden, and we all stand at the gate with the key. We just must learn how to open it and keep it from the weeds. And when the weeds do appear, learn how to eliminate them and take care of the rest of the garden.

Since Mark's death, I have had to learn how to laugh and enjoy life again. I have had to pick up the pieces and deal with the silence and hum in my head after the long drive on Caregiver Avenue. With all this though, I still try to weed and care for my garden when I can.

Mark's garden was full of so many wonderful things, his friends, his family, the nurses, the doctors, the people he worked with and all the caring people who helped him along the way. For someone who never planted anything in his life, he had the greenest thumb around when it came to his garden.

Since then, working with Homelessness, AIDS programs, the school system in Vermont, mental health programs and I am a board member for the Barre Community Justice Center. I was part of the group that created a camp for HIV affected families and the Opiate Response Team in Randolph VT which took the lead in about 2013 to fight the encroaching epidemic of opiate addiction. The house I live in is a 16 room Victorian that I hope to use as a respite for people affected by TBI. As you can see my garden is still growing and I feel blessed to be fortunate enough to do what I do.

My zest for living, learning and experiencing life has not changed, my energy level has changed quite a bit. I have found that even though I was under a lot of stress, had the occasional glass or glasses of wine, partied till wee hours in the morning and had two jobs for most of my life, I have learned how to live in moderation and focus on the things that matter. This can be very different for each of us. The Garden Gate, is a metaphor for the ability to tap into the important things that entertain or are meaningful in your life. The key can be as simple as the ability to choose a direction to go or a path to take in a life that can be so full of dead ends and potholes. You all have that ability, and it has taken me many years to come to that awakening.

My son has opened my eyes more than anything. If you have had your own kids, you will know what I mean. Even though he is not of my blood, the father/son relationship which has developed is stronger than ever. He was the key master in some ways that helped me open up the goodness in life that was just beyond the gate.

I have been lucky to have many key holders who showed me that I can open it up any time I want to. It is one of the most wonderful freedoms we have.

The garden can be as simple as a room where you can create your art if you are an artist, or the ability to work in the most amazing job ever, or a passion for the outdoors and the freedom to walk the wilderness at will. It can also be the freedom to take a nap in the afternoon or the opportunity to accomplish a dream long dreamed. These are some of the tools that make it real for me. Many of the victims of the holocaust I have met say that their garden was all in their mind. The horrors and fears that became the crossroads of life for them and shackled them to the pain of reality could have used a Garden that would be easily accessible in one's mind. To hear stories of their moments of sanity is quite amazing. Each garden is unique and personal. I hope you can find your key.

THE ANGER ZONE

After Mark and I knew what was happening medically and where we stood emotionally, we knew we were in for some bumpy roads ahead. It wasn't going to be easy to handle at times and there were going to be a lot of those potholes in the road. We knew so many people who had gone through similar experiences with caring for people with HIV. Some of the episodes we would recover from with little problem. It was the ones that we were not sure of that bothered us, and it would take longer emotionally to get through.

We decided to allow ourselves to show our anger or at least express it in some way and also show our compassion just as readily. The compassion, I felt, would be the hardest one because it is easier to recognize the anger and it is more visual and disruptive. This was to be one of the most important decisions we made at that point. When he could still walk, it was frustrating to see him in so much pain and be so angry but at least he was still walking and working. At work, he would spend most of his time behind the desk in the back with his leg up on something to keep the blood from throbbing in it. When he had a customer, he had to hold his pain in and watch what he said.

About a year before his death he was showing signs of weakening and would get tired very easily. For a while, he would come home from work and do his couch pillow on the floor routine and lie on the living room floor not wanting to eat or be bothered. I would sit on the couch with the TV on to keep me company. He would sleep restlessly through the night, get up, take a shower and get dressed. I would take him to work and go about my daily chores. I was only working freelance at the time, so I had a lot of time to do the things I thought I needed to do. I would call in on the hour to see how he was and then pick him up after work. He would only eat if he thought he could keep it down. That wasn't often so I made sure he had his vitamins and supplements as often as I could. Then the routine would begin all over again.

One evening I couldn't sleep. I kept my mind off the situation by watching TV. One of the programs on that night at about 1:00 AM was called the Psychic Network, a show dedicated to the idea that there were other levels in life and death most of us could not comprehend. My father believed there was a supernatural world and was often in contact with local psychics on WKRI radio station in Rhode Island. Allowing my curiosity to carry me, I listened to the program while one person after another gave testimony to their beliefs and experiences with psychics. Much of it sounded rehearsed, and I am sure it was. But remembering how my father spoke of his experiences with it, I listened on.

Being desperate for something to entertain me and remembering that dad had told me it never hurts to try to find out if it is for me, I decided to call. I felt a little silly doing it and after I got the phone bill a little guilty, not to mention broke. Those calls do cost a lot of money. The person I spoke to told me some things which, at first, didn't make sense. One was that Nellie and Joe were two of my guardian angels who were watching me all the time. She asked me if I knew who they were. I couldn't think of anyone in my past who was dead who might be my guardian angel with those names. Also, she said I would be taking a trip in late fall to a cold and grey place. I would travel over a large body of water alone to do something wonderful. I had no plans to go anywhere and with Mark feeling the way he did I could not think of anything else but taking care of him.

After I hung up, I thought about some of the things she had said. Many of them were on the money like him saying that I was concerned about my father who had heart problems and that my camera was one of the tools that would keep my mind off the stress. He also said my mother was around me all the time and that was why I think of her often. I did think of her every day but I couldn't figure out who Nellie and Joe were. I got up off the couch to see how Mark was and got ready to go to sleep. I spent a lot of time sleeping on the couch in the living room just so I could be there if Mark needed me for something.

Later that week I was telling one of my friends what the psychic had said. After explaining it all, she asked me if any of my relatives had those names. I thought back as far as I could. Then it hit me. My grandmother's name was Nellie, but we were used to calling her Gram. Also, her first husband, my biological grandfather, was Joseph and Gram used to call him Joe sometimes. It was one of those ah-ha moments to be sure.

A few weeks later I received a call from Jacque who I had met previously. He bought the Christmas animation from B. Altman's department store after they went out of business. He hired me in the spring of 1991 to dismantle the displays and crate them up so he could take them to Poland. There he owned a company called Multi-Investment International. It had been almost a year since I had heard from him and I thought I had seen the last of him at that time. His call was a complete surprise.

"I need you to come to Poland to set up the displays in my new stores. I want you to reconstruct them here the way they looked in New York. I will make it worth your while," he said. I told him that I would have to think it over as there was something I would have to deal with here and I would let him know.

Mark had been feeling much better, as he was taking new medicine and going to the gym regularly. This was one of those high points on that roller coaster people refer to sometimes. He seemed like he was out of the woods for the time being. This made it easier to decide about going to Poland. It looked as if he was well on his way to recovery from his previous condition. I asked him if he would be all right for a week or two on his own. He agreed that this was an opportunity I should not miss, and I should go for it. I knew he was scared, but he assured me he would be OK.

The Psychic was right. I left in November for Poland, a place I had only heard and read about from stories of World War II. The day came when I had to leave, and he helped me with the packing and preparing myself mentally for this new adventure. He could drive, but I insisted that a friend take him and me to the airport so he would not have to drive back alone. He agreed. The airport scene was a tough one. We had not been separated for this long except when we moved to Connecticut. I could see he was nervous about me going away as I was his primary Caregiver. But for the two weeks, he held it together well. He wasn't one to show his emotions in public. We said our goodbyes and I was off.

Arriving in Warsaw on a cloudy day at the airport was an experience I won't soon forget. The airport terminal was not very big and not well taken care of. Surrounding the building was an army of uniformed men with military rifles as if guarding a monument.

I got through customs and met the people who were to drive me to their office. On the way, I couldn't help but notice that everything was so grey, I assumed a result of the former communist government. Being winter, the trees had no leaves, and the ground was bare. The buildings were all the same stone grey, and the people wore dark or light grey, simple clothing. I felt like I was in a black and white movie.

The next day I began my work by getting everything ready to set up the windows in the store that faced the square called Plaza Constituski which I believe means Constitution Square. This was reportedly one of the squares where Lech Walesa spoke to his followers and gave a liberation speech. Later that week I would stay in the hotel where he delivered the speech from the balcony facing the square. While setting up the windows, I met some of the people who would be helping me. Only one of them spoke English which made him my translator. When he was not around it was like a comedy routine. It was like pulling teeth to get them to do or understand what had to be done. At one point, I got very frustrated and was ready to give it all up.

Someone had mentioned that this work crew likes beer. I recall several of the workers inviting me to go for a few drinks a couple of times, but I had to keep at the windows if I was to finish them by the deadline. I decided to put a carrot in front of the horse so to speak. I tried to explain to them what had to be done in a sort of a primitive sign language to no avail. Finally I was able to get in touch with the guy who spoke English and asked him to tell them that if we could get the platforms up and the wiring was complete, I would buy them the beer.

The platforms were done in short order, the wiring was finished, and we even got some of the partitions in place. It was now Miller time, or whatever the beer was called. They didn't get paid much, about $10.00 American per day, but for the beer it was worth it. The rest of the week went like clockwork, and they even brought their friends to help those who were not on the payroll.

My thoughts of Mark were constant, and I worried he was not feeling well. I called him several times, which was good for both of us, yet it was difficult in so many ways. I wanted to be with him, but I wanted to be in Poland also.

While I was working in the windows, many of the local people came walking by to see what was going on. The colors and animation fascinated the children. It was as if they were in a wide-eyed trance. The elderly people were showing a sense of nostalgia or relief that their Christmas spirit was about to come back. It had been many years since they had seen anything like this. But it was the middle-aged people born during or just after the war who showed mistrust and a sense that something was not right. Standing stern-faced with their arms crossed, they spelled defiance and fear. They had lived under strict Communism for most, if not all of their lives and the change was skeptically welcome.

At the end of the week, I was witness to one of the first Christmas celebrations to be held in a public square in over 45 years. A tree, not unlike the one in New York at Rockefeller Center was erected and decorated with live angels descending from the top by a crane, singing to the crowds and illuminated by searchlights giving a shimmering effect to their costumes. I arrived in a limo with Jacque. I later learned that the limo was one of the only stretch limos in Warsaw. I was allowed free-roaming privileges in front of the ropes with my camera and attended the party held later with all the delegates and representatives from all over the world which was held in the old presidential palace, now a museum.

While watching the ceremony, I recall seeing the children and enjoying their looks of wonder. There had to be several thousand people in the huge square who were standing in the cold to see this wonderful event. It was the children's eyes that got me and the tears from the adults that made me feel proud and lucky that I was an American and living in a free country, something I had taken for granted quite frequently. The people of this area were very resilient as I learned that the whole area including the original Palace was destroyed by the Nazis in World War II. From the pictures, I have seen since my visit I realize now what strength and pride they had. To have to live under a communist government which restricted many of the freedoms we seldom think about and take for granted. The area was completely reconstructed to its original state from pictures and documents that survived the war. Yet to walk down the streets, you would think it was built in the 1700s.

That night I called Mark and told him how wonderful it all was. I sensed he was not feeling well, but he tried to cover it up. I decided to cut my stay short and come home. I didn't know what this illness had in store for Mark or myself as his Caregiver and couldn't deal with being there for him long-distance anymore.

I had experienced one of the most memorable events I will ever have ever witnessed. Now it was time to come home. Mark was looking thinner, but he was still healthy considering all he was going through. I also knew he had broken one of the rules we had agreed upon. He held in his anger about me going away while he was ill so I could take advantage of the trip of a lifetime. I forgave him but was angry he held it in. We talked about it a while and agreed that it wasn't healthy to hold in the anger. We vowed never to do it again. So much for vows.

There were times when it was not realistic to admit to being angry, but we knew we were doing it and that made the difference.

I was scheduled to go back to Poland in February and do some more work on the windows. I had kept the number of a psychic I had called earlier. I wanted to see what she would have to say about the trip in February. She did not know my name or where I was from only that I called her once before. I don't know how she could have remembered who I was. When I was talking to her, I asked about the trip in February which would occur the first week of the month and how things would work out.

She told me I would be traveling over a body of water, not in the first week but the second. I hadn't received any notice of a change, but I let her go on. She said it would be a very relaxing place where I would meet new friends. It would also be warm and pleasant. I wasn't sure, but I didn't think that Poland was anywhere near warm in February. I asked her if it was Poland I was going to. She said that it was south of where I was now and that she didn't see me going to Poland at all.

I had no plans to go south and even tried to find out if any relatives or friends were going to get married in February who might be from the south. I would still have to go over a body of water she said, and the only place I knew that I would have any friends to visit was Brazil where I lived for over a year.

I had to put it out of my mind, or I would go crazy. With Christmas over, the decorations now in their boxes, the skeletal remains of dry abandoned Christmas Trees now lined the roads. Their short moment of glory, now forgotten as if it were a faded dream meant that I now had to start to think about spring. I tried to get in touch with Jacque in Poland to finish up the loose ends. I spoke to him once which was not the most encouraging conversation as he was not sure how things would pan out concerning the economic situation in his country. His last words to me were "I will let you know."

I began to wonder about the psychic and what she had told me. Mark had been feeling pretty good and was now suffering from cabin fever. With the weather so cold it was getting risky for him to be outside. One evening while we were eating, he said he wanted to go somewhere to get away for awhile. He had looked at a lot of places in the travel section of the papers and had decided he wanted to go to Cancun. With his sense of urgency, it was as if he felt it would be his last chance to go anywhere.

The thought of this being his last chance to have the opportunity to go away hit home. I don't know what it was like for him to know this. I could only imagine what it would have been like for me and that was not a pleasant thought. There was a part of me that thought he might have been jealous of me having traveled so much out of the country. As a Caregiver, I had to put on my smiley face and go with it. Yet deep down inside, I was worried.

Mark, being the planner and organizer that he was, went to the travel agent to make all the arrangements. The least expensive time to go was the second week in February. It was also one of the more comfortable times in Mexico where the weather was not too hot, meaning not over 90 degrees. When he told me the plans, I remembered what the psychic had said about going the second week instead of the first which was to be my trip to Poland. I began to think that this psychic stuff could get addictive, let alone expensive. Luckily it didn't, and in fact, I would rather not know how things are going to turn out most of the time, as much as my curiosity tempts me.

Mark's inability to tolerate little things that bothered him was growing, and there were some flare-ups before we went, but I was glad he was getting it out in the open and dealing with it. He had been going to the hospital for radiation treatments about twice a week, and he wasn't sure if the trip would interrupt any progress. The doctor told him to go and have a good time. He had asked the doctor if he could take a vacation from the medication. The answer was simple, not advisable. But Mark being Mark, he was afraid that if they searched his luggage, they would find them and he would be labeled. The cat out of the bag, so to speak. He put them in an aspirin bottle, but I also think he did not take them when he should have. By doing this it would allow the virus to accelerate faster. I would soon see him getting sicker at a more rapid pace, and yet I did not want to attribute his actions.

So off to Cancun, it was. The plane was a nightmare, and the seats were so close together; there was no room for stretching his legs. He had developed some spots on his leg, which were diagnosed as Kaposi's Sarcoma. They were high enough on his leg that he could wear shorts and they would not show. This became an issue as he knew people would react to the spots and make judgments on him, especially at home, when he went to the gym and took a shower, or used the steam room. Also, his legs were beginning to swell. The spot on his leg was now appropriately named "Spot."

While we were in Cancun, things were going well. He was happy and enjoying the sights and the sun. This was the first time he had gone to another country, so he wanted everything to be perfect. We decided to take one of the side trips to see the Mayan Ruins. Of course, we picked the hottest day, but it was all worth it.

When we got to the first ruin, being the photographer I was, I felt I wanted to shoot everything in sight. I still didn't have it in my head yet that this was going to be his last vacation. I guess I didn't want to. He had to take it slow as he was getting tired easily. When we got to the top of the biggest one, he became nervous, so he went down before me while I spent a little more time shooting. I thought I had my eye on him, but I lost sight of him. I think he might have gone out of sight to teach me a lesson. I frantically looked for him, hoping he was OK. Thoughts of failing as a Caregiver came to the surface. When I finally met up with him, I could see his anger bubbling. We both said things we would regret and we hurt each other's feelings, but we said them, and there was no turning back. They were brutal words. I was now an inconsiderate, selfish son of a bitch who did not give a damn whether he lived or died. He was now a selfish little spoiled invalid who only cares about himself. We exchanged some bad vibes yet I knew why they were said. This was his trip, and it had to be special. He knew deep down inside that it was probably his last one. I also needed a vacation or some space but, again that truth about being the Caregiver had shown its ugly face. I am in his world, and my world comes second.

At the time, I didn't know or see how much he needed to share his experience totally with me while he was still here breathing, thinking and dreaming. I guess we all get a little selfish at times. When we become selfish, we lose sight of each other's needs. We sat down and talked it over on one of the sacrificial altars. We were both sacrificing something of ourselves for the other. Where we were, seemed symbolically appropriate. For the first time, I saw in his eyes the fear and hatred toward this invisible enemy called AIDS.

I had finally opened my eyes and my heart during that brief moment. For the first time, we were talking to each other through our hearts and not our egos. We agreed that there would be more arguments, but it was OK because of what came after the yelling and harsh words. A base of true understanding was what I saw. This would carry us through some pretty hard times to come.

We knew we were in the "anger zone". It was a place we had heard about and thought we were prepared for. We weren't though. What I didn't know then was that I would carry the anger right through to the present. I still get angry with AIDS and what it has taken from me over the years. But now I only show it with people who care, and at times I direct it towards them without even knowing I am doing it. I used to apologize all the time for being angry, but most of my friends know what it is and where it comes from. Most of them can usually handle it. Directing it elsewhere used to be the only outlet I knew of to release the anger. Of course, there are a few people I get angry with who I feel deserve it. They are people who try to help or intrude to the point of smothering. They might use the phrase, "You should be over this by now." Some of them don't know when to stop, and fortunately, I have taken steps to delete them from my life. I can't talk to them as they still can't acknowledge that they have done anything. Moving, changing my telephone number and not being home much, were for a while the only way to stop it outside of a court order. There is only one person

I show my anger to who understands and receives my anger willingly. He respects the fact that at times I need to vent it in a way where I can get a positive response. For years it was my long time friend Sal but he was in RI. For a while I had no one until one day I met this guy at a social event in town. He had lost his partner and could relate to what I was going through. His name was Patric. A huge burly guy with the arms of a weightlifter. We went out for drinks one night and he said that if I ever needed to punch something to just call him. I called him a few weeks later and he said to meet him at the Episcopal Church. When I walked into the office it became obvious he was a minister. An Irish Episcopal priest. I jokingly refer to him as my God sent. We all need that one person.

Since then I have found that the emotion "anger" is so important in the healing process. Expressing it is even more important. Yet I still have a hard time letting it go, which causes me more pain and at times more anger. Mark and I went through so much that I rarely like to bring it up for fear of bringing up tears and memories.

There was another time when anger overwhelmed us both. We had just put a hospital bed in the room Mark was sleeping in. I felt Mark would be more comfortable there and he wouldn't have to move as the bed was adjustable. The day had gone quietly with Mark cat napping most of the day. I had just made a meal and was cleaning the dishes out of the room. He pointed to the blinds in the window and insisted that they were not level. I lowered them until they were to his satisfaction. He then told me to move some books off the table and straighten out the bedsheets. I then put the pillow under his foot to raise it a little higher. At that point, I was furious. I felt like throwing the books, dishes and the world at him. I left the room slamming the door, but not saying anything. A few minutes later I came back to apologize to him.

He then said, "What is the matter with you? You know I need help." At this point, we were yelling at each other, and again things were said we would later regret.

With tears in our eyes, he continued, "Do you know what it is like to know I won't be here much longer and will have to leave you alone?"

I answered, "Do you know what it is like for me to know that you might not be here much longer and I'll have to go on by myself?"

It was that moment we both understood each other's pain. We were afraid to leave each other. I never saw him cry in front of someone. We made a vow, (yes, another vow), that we would learn to tolerate each other's anxiety and work with it. We still had to express our anger, but tolerance was the key. It had been ten years that day since we first met, or at least as close as we could figure. Seeing him cry for the first time made that moment a milestone.

Watching him die was not my idea of a fun day at the park, but I had to be there for him. Right about then he asked me if it would be all right if his mother came to stay with him for a few days at a time. I didn't know her well except for a brief meeting at the hospital and through phone conversations concerning his health. I knew his time was growing short and was sure he also knew this. I called his mother, and we spoke for some time. I wanted to let her know how important it was to him and myself for her to be there. She was more than welcome to stay as long as she wanted. The days she was there gave us valuable time to connect as friends. Mark could see this and loved every minute of it, even when he complained. I could see his mom holding in a lot. One afternoon I saw her in the kitchen. Mark was asleep. I could see she had been crying and gave her a hug. Suddenly she started pounding my chest and gritting her teeth. She said she was so angry but could not tell Mark. I let her pound away and we sat and talked for close to an hour.

Again, I saw how important anger was to all of us and that expressing it helped us understand each other as if it were a time out from normality. We didn't know it, but the weeks to follow would be the toughest for all of us. Our preparation and training so to speak would be the guide that would help us through and allow ourselves to acknowledge our feelings. I can't say it works 100 % but I can say it helped us get through some of the hard times.

I see now that we can't always jump into situations like this and use crisis intervention, although much of my life has been lived like this. We sometimes must go one step at a time to allow ourselves to heal and be healed by others' compassion and actions. I am glad I had the opportunity to feel these feelings of anger and at times rage. I hope that when a time of anger comes again, I will remember.

SOMEBODY'S HERO

It was July, hot and sticky. There was only one air conditioner in the house, and it was in Mark's room. Because it was there the door had to be closed, so his connection to the outside world was now limited to the television and the many trips to the doctor. We had just gone through an episode of getting him in and out of the tub. A nice warm bath was one of the things that would give him a few moments of peace.

He could still use his crutches and did so when going from the tub to the bed. One thing I began to notice was that when he sat or stood up, he would begin to panic and say that his stomach was being crushed. I would find out later that his body and lungs were filling up with fluid at such a rapid rate that it would eventually have to be extracted.

The Connecticut Forum on AIDS was on one of the local channels. They seemed to be bickering back and forth about a lot of issues dealing with HIV/AIDS, housing, funding for treatment and a host of other issues which were forefront in the minds of the community, nation and the world. They showed a clip of Arthur Ashe, telling in his own words the fight he was fighting. Mark had a great deal of admiration for Arthur and was listening intently. We two were in on the conversation, enclosed by the safety of his four walls. He was amazed to see Mr. Ashe speak about his situation so freely and not feel the fear of discrimination he felt just going to work. It was not right. Mark would say several times that we can spend billions of dollars on guns, ammunition and military personnel to fight and kill in the name of protecting our assets and can't find the few million dollars to fight for saving the lives of millions who are HIV positive. He saw it as a moral judgment that the people who could help seeing people who were positive as responsible for their illness as if to say, "you got it you deal with it". In part, he felt they were right that he had made choices without having that crystal ball to allow him to become aware of the consequences. Yet when people smoke to the point of getting cancer, that is acceptable enough to provide millions of dollars to the research of finding a cure or a drug that would end the pain of cancer. They were making choices also. And what about the thousands who got it through blood transfusions? Did that make it more acceptable or in his words, "morally comfortable to deal with?"

We could have gone on and on. About ten minutes after the clip was over, a man came to the mic and said, "There is something I have to do, and I don't know if I can, so I have to ask a few people to stand by me." There was a long silence. Then, he continued, "What I have to say is so inappropriate and yet so appropriate…" He paused. "Arthur Ashe was admitted to a hospital a few minutes ago."

The silence that followed was deafening. Nothing was said for a few minutes. Mark's face was still. He looked at me and gave me a hug. I could see him looking at his own illness progressing. I knew what he was feeling, but couldn't sense the intensity of it. The rest of the day was a very slow, hot July day. I was so relieved when it ended. That night, going to bed, I felt a sense of relief I will never forget.

Mark would sleep in intervals. I was awake for most of the day, but at night when he was wide awake and in pain, he would let me sleep. It was like a daily payment for putting up with his demands and pain. He also said I snore.

He found his hero. Someone who was intent on letting people know what was happening. Someone who gave himself the opportunity to make a difference. The next day, Mark asked me to sit next to him so we could talk. One of the statements he made is still stuck in my mind. It's one of the main reasons why I wrote this book. He said, "Of all the things I have done in my life I have only one regret that haunts me. That regret is that I never gave myself the chance to make a difference."

I wanted to knock some sense into him and tell him what a difference he has made in my life and so many others. I just didn't know how.

He had once said that he thought of doing something with his spare time to help others, or work with Boy Scout groups or something that would give him a sense of doing something good. That hot steamy July I found my hero. One who made all the difference in the world. Mark.

February 6, 1993, I was sitting with friends watching an old Arthur Ashe speech. The program was interrupted by a news bulletin saying that Arthur Ashe died earlier in his hospital room. We all knew Mark looked up to him and one of us said, "now they can chat it up."

THE PICNIC

The day was warm, a bit humid but pleasant. The snow was just about completely melted, leaving only a patchwork of white and brownish-green. It was one of those first days of spring you pray for during the cold and rainy episodes of late winter. I called some of Mark's friends to ask them if they wanted to have a small picnic. Several of them agreed, and we were off. The place was a favorite of Mark's where he used to go to sit quietly and think. Around the pond, there were stone benches where he could sit while he fed the ducks and geese.

We sat under the tree, which was now beginning to bud next to his stone marker. Yes, it was the cemetery where he was buried. One of Mark's favorite songs was "With a Little Help from My Friends" which was inscribed on his grave marker. I had often visited the spot to listen to myself a bit and get over the tragedy and wonder of his death. We sat around nervously wondering if what we were doing was OK. The conversation was light, and we were just taking in the warmth of the day.

Most of the conversations were memories of days with Mark, which helped us feel better about being there. We cleared the winter debris from the area. It was like we had to do something constructive to justify our presence. The blanket and wreath we had put there for the Christmas Season were still frozen in place. We brought a few apples and some sandwiches to munch on, but we all felt there was a little lunacy about having a picnic in a graveyard.

Some words were said, and then they were all off to do whatever they had to do that day. I stayed behind. It is often hard to say things at a grave, as you feel like someone might see you and think you are losing it. I began to think, "can he really hear or understand what I am saying, or is this just for my benefit?" Memories of all the good times we had flooded my mind. I tried to fill him in on what was happening in my life as if I was talking to him face to face.

I thought of how hard it had been for both of us while he was sick, and felt the tears begin to well up. You know that stage of emotion where you need to cry, but you hold it back? That is where I was. It was so hard to accept what happened and yet there was a lot of good through it all. I told him how difficult it had been for his family and me without him any longer. But standing there and sharing all my words, I felt he knew what I was thinking, and I began to clean up some of the twigs that had fallen from the tree around his grave.

Some geese came up from the pond and I gave them part of my sandwich. It took my mind off the sadness I was feeling, along with the mixed emotions. I decided to take a walk around the pond and see where he mentioned visiting on several occasions. I saw the stone benches that were grave markers surrounding the pond and inscribed with names and dates. Knowing how he loved the beach and especially the ocean, I could understand that he would sit here next to this motionless body of water except for an occasional incoming duck or goose. Water in any quantity can be a soothing source of peace and calm. I sat on one of the benches and thought of all the days I spent caring for Mark. They were hard days, but they made me strong and gave me a new awareness I had not known.

The brisk yet warm air had a cleansing effect on me, helping me to think more about what I had gone through in the past year. For the first time, I began to feel like things were going to be alright. The pond, geese and the quiet of the area gave me solace and helped me realize how important it was for me to relax and take time out for me. It was like Mark was there leading me around by the hand, showing me his special spot.

It was getting late, and I had a lot to do. I went back to the gravesite and said a prayer thanking Mark for all he did for me, and I hope that he is in a safe place with no pain. I began packing some of the tools I brought out to clean around the grave-a rake, a spade and a few baskets full of debris. I didn't want to leave, but I knew that if I stayed much longer it would make it more difficult to leave. While packing the car, I ran across a couple of things Mark had left in the trunk. I thought to myself as I held back a tear, will it ever get easier? And if it does, will I feel guilty about that?

Ready to go, I touched the grave one last time. I don't know why, but you see it in the movies when a loved one passes. It was like that stone was the closest I could get to him. I looked at the grave and said, "Good-bye, my friend" which was also the title of a song by Yanni, that Mark had said he liked. I could never find it, but I would keep looking. I walked to the car as I watched the geese retreat from feasting on my sandwiches. Opening the car door, I turned and looked one more time, still silent. As I glanced upward I saw the little birdhouse his father had hung from the tree, swinging in the soft, warm, welcome breeze. I watched it and said to myself, "Today was a gift from Mark." It was a wonderful and welcome gift.

Suddenly I felt the urge to go, as if Mark were saying "Enough already." I got in, started the car and went quietly. I don't think I have ever driven so slow. Reaching the gate to the cemetery, my foot hit the gas pedal, and I was off to continue my day.

On the way home, my mind began to wander. I thought about the day when I found out he was HIV positive. I had taken the train from Grand Central Station in New York to Glenbrook in Stamford many times but that day was a little different. I felt something was about to happen. I didn't know what it was or if it was good or bad. It was just something.

I sat in the window seat, which is what I try to do whenever I take the train or plane as it gives me a sort of different dimension with which to think. Being in a visual profession I enjoy the sensation of the trees passing as the train plunges on. If I am sitting looking at the back of the train, sort of seeing where I have been, it becomes almost therapeutic, almost as if all the stress of the day's events are being sucked out of my being and hurled away from me to the back of the train.

The train has become a tranquilizing or calming agent for me. I usually daydream when riding the train. I seem to do most of my creative thinking in this mode, but this time was different. I began to experience every type of emotion from joy to panic.

About two earlier, I had spoken to Mark on the phone. He had been losing weight and not feeling well and went to the doctor that morning for a checkup. His voice on the phone was distant, yet to the point and positive. After a brief conversation about what he might do that evening, he added, "There is something I have to tell you that is going to make a big difference in our lives and how we do things. Please, come right home. I will see you then." Then he hung up with no good-bye, which he never did. I was usually the first to hang up. I later found out he had been crying. The quick end to our conversation was because he was afraid he would break down while we were talking.

I tried to look on the bright side. I thought of every positive thing that could make a difference in my life. Money, my tax refund, a new apartment, a job offer, winning the lottery, just anything that could change my life or make it better would have been nice. Everything that came to my mind peaked my imagination.

The train took an hour to get to Glenbrook from New York City. My mind spent 90% of it in another dimension. As the train approached Glenbrook station, I began to think about negative things. I began to get scared. I took my time getting home, which was only a ten-minute walk from the station. I stopped at the deli, which marked the halfway point between the station and my apartment, where I got my usual buttered roll and coffee. Not a healthy choice, but one I cherished and enjoyed. I stopped to talk to the two guys who owned the deli, who were behind the counter. After a minute or two I realized I was in a strange state of mind and that I should be going. They were always people I could talk to. They both had a funny, friendly way about themselves. They loved to make puns and jokes. One of them even saved me one day when my car wouldn't start by lending me his truck to jump the car. They were really friendly people.

It was time to confront my worst fears. So, I bolted out the door of the deli and ran up the embankment adjacent to my street spilling my coffee as I jumped the guard rail at the top. Our apartment was at the other end of the bridge which passed over the New Haven Railroad. If you looked out my living room window, you could see most of the bridge and the embankment at the side of the road. Upset, I ran for awhile and then stopped to catch my breath. I decided to slow down to a walk so that if Mark is watching, he wouldn't see me running. You could hear the train whistle from my apartment, so he could have conceivably been waiting to see if I was on my way or what was taking so long.

When I got to the door, I stopped. I took a deep breath. As I put the key into the keyhole, the door flew open, scraping my knuckles on the casing. I came face to face with my downstairs neighbor or "Warden" as he was known among the other tenants. Mark didn't get along with him, as he had a habit of telling everyone what they were doing wrong and keeping guard over the apartments. That was OK except when friends came to the house. They were always approached by him and told they couldn't park in the lot, or they were to close or far away from the lines designated for parking. I could usually understand his concerns even though he was a little overprotective of the place, but this time his concerns were the furthest from my mind.

As I stood there trying to get my key out of the door, he began to tell me that Mark had parked too far over the line in the parking lot and Mark wouldn't answer the phone or the door. Telling him I would handle it, as I usually did to get him off my back, I climbed the stairs taking two steps at a time. He mumbled something and slammed the door. I got the key in the door to the apartment at the top of the stairs and opened it slowly. All the lights were out, and the rooms were darkened as the sun had just set.

I walked into the living room and saw Mark on the couch with his head at the far end and his feet propped up at the end closest to me. He had sort of a half-smile on his face and asked me to sit next to him a minute. He started by saying, "I don't know quite how to tell you and don't know how you will take what I have to say." He stopped for a moment as if to build courage. "I have AIDS," he said. "I went to the doctor and got my results. They came back positive for HIV."

There was a long silence. I felt helpless, strong and afraid, all at the same time. I was speechless.

"Say something," he said.

"Say what?" I said.

"I don't know, hate me, yell at me, tell me off, scream, love me, I don't know," he said.

The silence that came next was so loud it was deafening to me. I could hear my heart beating.

Finally, a few words were said and we began to talk about our friendship and the time we had left together rather than think in terms of finality. We knew each day and each moment would be important from that moment on. As we spoke, I thought how much different our lives might have been if we had lived this philosophy. I began to feel guilty a bit that I hadn't lived each day to the fullest. Then I felt guilty about feeling guilty. We both knew it was going to be rough. We also knew there would be some upsets, but they had to be handled when we got to them. The main thing that came out of this was that he was so relieved to find out that I was not going to move out or reject his condition. I told him that our friendship was stronger than any illness.

We decided to change our dialogue to be more positive. When someone mentioned dying with AIDS, we changed it to living with AIDS. Many of the "if"s were changed to "when"s. We decided to learn as much about each other as possible, especially each other's needs. As friends it was important, but more so for me as his Caregiver. It was all a learning process, but there was no teacher. AIDS did not come with an instruction book. We knew from having met other Caregivers and people who were HIV positive that it was going to be a wild ride.

Even though the dialogue was good and upbeat, I still felt like we were in a canoe without a paddle, floating at the will of the river. I had no idea where to start. I just knew I had to start. We both had to look at everything realistically. When reports in the news spoke of "Hope" on TV and in the papers, we had to read "Hope" and not promise. There were so many "if" and not enough "when"s. Just the same, we had to make it all work for us.

Someone told me shortly after I learned that Mark was diagnosed positive for HIV, "When someone becomes ill, more than one suffers." I wasn't sure how I would fit into that at first, but I quickly learned. I was aware early on that I had to take as much care of myself as I was taking care of Mark, if not more.

The doctor told Mark he had to start eating healthy and working out regularly. He also told him that my part in the illness would be different from his, but just as debilitating at times on an emotional level. He was referring to stress and depression accompanied by exhaustion. A good vitamin program would be appropriate for both of us. I spoke to my doctor about what I should be taking, and his suggestion was vitamin B12, C, D, and a lot of antioxidants. He also said to consider juicing vegetables and fruits.

In this light, we worked out a schedule of how and when we would do as much of the vitamin regime and how we could do it together for support. Mark didn't want to bring any more people into the picture just yet. It would bother him that others were at risk of stress, etc. I agreed, up to a point. I did tell my family because I felt I was going to need their support. This support came in the form of just asking how he and I were, which helped me not feel alone for the most part.

I felt it was important that some dialog happened on the outside, so to speak. Experiencing something of this nature on your own can be a horrible experience. The anxiety it can cause can be devastating. For about a year, we struggled to make it all work. My schedule was tight and full of things I felt were important at the time, my job as visual merchandiser, friends, my commitment to making sure we had food, gas, etc. Then without warning, I lost my job. I nearly lost my mind. "What am I going to do now?" came out of my mouth often. I was desperately afraid. But when Mark said, "Don't worry, we will work it out," somehow that made it OK. Mark had always been one to be in control, and if things didn't go well, his anger would show. He was a planner and a budget wizard and could balance a checkbook in minutes. Being HIV positive became a big threat to him, as it took away a bit of his control. This time was different. He understood how hard it was for me to lose my job. He began to feel helpless, yet he became my support system and cheerleader. We truly became our brother's keeper.

During that year I began to see a lot of hate and prejudice from the community associated with the illness. With people not knowing the position I was in, they would say what was on their mind and give their opinions freely. I remember one day I was sitting in a diner. A woman began to speak quite loudly. There had been something on the TV above the bar about AIDS. She responded by saying, "We should put all the 'AIDS people' on an island and blow it up. Then we wouldn't have to worry about it anymore. Besides, they are all faggots anyway." That sounded like the attitude our government had in the early eighties. My response to her was, "They are not the ones we should worry about," meaning she was more dangerous to society than all her faggots. She didn't quite understand what I meant and shrugged her shoulders while she finished her coffee.

I knew then I had to learn how to be more selfish. I had to take care of my things and Mark's things first, or neither of us were going to make it. It became more and more evident that I was now Mark's Caregiver. I read as much about AIDS as I could. I learned relaxation methods that I still use today. A friend of mine, who was a psychologist in Massachusetts and worked with me at the group home in Andover, helped me through my mother's death, along with the help of the residents of the group home. He introduced me to some relaxation tapes and exercises. If I hadn't had them, I don't know if I would have come through it all the way I did.

I found music could help my state of relaxation, so I focused on it. Most of the work of Yanni had been a welcome part of my life. In the summer, I would take my Walkman and relax on the beach in town, listening to music and the waves. This became one of my lifesavers.

There were times I couldn't tell Mark I was at the beach as he would say things like "What is more important, me or the beach?" It is so hard to defend yourself in this situation with someone who is in pain all the time. I felt that if I didn't give myself some time out, I wouldn't be able to handle what was to come.

It seemed funny how certain songs stuck in my head that meant something or were related to what we were going through. One song still affects me when I hear it. Peter Gabriel did a song called "Don't Give Up" which summed up a lot for me during this time and gave me a sense of strength. Later it was Eric Clapton's "Tears in Heaven" and Elton John's "Father and Son." I sometimes felt they were singing those songs to me, Mark and my father as I was dealing with my father's illness and death at the same time as I was going through this with Mark. My dad died in March, and Mark died in July of the same year.

With all this death in such a short time, I was looking for support in some form. A friend of mine told me there was a support group around for people who have lost someone with AIDS. I was reluctant to join, but finally decided it was time to look into it. This group became very helpful in helping me not feel alone. One of the sessions began with a woman who spoke about her problems dealing with their child's illness. It was a story to beat all stories,(not that we were in competition in this support group), but it was a tough one to speak of and just as tough to listen to. She, like most of us, was looking for some answers to questions which could only be answered in time. But listening to her helped me feel like I was not in this alone, but together with many players who needed to express their feelings.

While hearing her story, I remembered getting ready for "the big one" so to speak. I felt like I was preparing for a hurricane which is so unpredictable no one knows just how to prepare for it except education and guts. We must be educated and ready for the worst. The one thing I suggested to do was do what a friend did. When he knew that it was going to be hard for him to offer help, he just prepared himself and told me that he would be there whenever Mark or I needed him. The day came, and our pride was swallowed partly by exhaustion. Between doctor visits, medicine, and every emotional ride we were both at the end of our emotional and physical limits. He was there for us and stayed to the end. He and others came through with flying colors. But it was all about timing. To them, I extend my eternal thanks.

I think we cannot try to be heroes or saviors in this situation. There are too many factors involved, whether they be political or social, religious or spiritual, confidentiality or dignity. There are so many facets to this stone that being the hero or savior will only cause another facet to fail or affect many other facets in a negative way. I look back at the days and nights I took care of Mark and only remember seeing myself on automatic. I did whatever had to be done at the moment and tried to save the emotions for tougher times.

My biggest fears were that Mark's family would not acknowledge the magnitude of our friendship, along with the stereotypes of AIDS. I had those doubts right up to the end. You tend to overhear people's remarks and stay silent in times like these. When Mark's father came up to me at the funeral and saw my hesitant behavior, he put his arm around my neck and said, "None of this crap. You are family. You belong up front in the receiving line with the rest of us." Frank, our best friend and former roommate, saw this happening and decided to make himself an honorary family member and stayed up there with us. I know why he did it and was glad he did. It did ease the tension and lighten up the moment.

That all blew me away. I had to step back a minute and pull myself together, as it was like receiving an award of acknowledgment for just being a good friend and Caregiver. I never expected to hear that, even though I knew there were different levels of acceptance in the family. The acceptance was still there. Losing my father four months before and having only my sister as my family at Mark's funeral was a feeling I could never express to them. I also felt that the time Mark's mother and I spent together while Mark was still in the hospital bed at home would be the beginning of a great relationship, or at least I was hoping at the time. I didn't have to look to them for help. They were there for me without boundaries. You could almost say unconditionally. The relationship was unlimited. There were no spoken rules, but there was a lot of trust. I only wish that Mark was around to see this all unfold. I'm sure he was watching. It seems sad that so many times in life it takes a death or tragedy to create an outpouring of love, acceptance and new awareness without judgment. I wouldn't feel that again until 9/11 when the Trade Towers fell. It was not as personal except for the fact that I had a bit of a connection to the Towers and knew a few people there, but it was a little different. I feel lucky. I know of so many situations where it got worse rather than better. The relatives, friends, and partners of those who were HIV positive were left with no will and to abandon all they had done for someone they loved and because of stigma and society they had to act as if it all never happened. Sometimes family members would insist on gaining possession of many material things that may have been a part of the deceased life but connected to a friend or partner, female or male, that not only has monetary value but also sentimental value. I have seen this cold wind blow. I do feel lucky that a lot of what he and I had collected together as friends were left up to me to distribute and not at the hands of vultures.

I have found that judgment of one another, AIDS-related or not, creates barriers and defenses which will separate and keep people from seeing the true joy that can be had in a friendship or any relationship. Just look at racism in America and around the world. Who will forget the greatest hate crime in recent history, Hitler and his henchmen? Now after all the opportunities to learn from our mistakes we have had Bosnia, Darfur, and Iraq as well as many more unmentioned.

Unfortunately, judgments will be around as long as there are two different people standing on this earth. The potential is there. There were some days when Mark was sick that I saw evil all around. Those days made the good days look better.

I want to share something that happened in December which came to my mind while sitting on the bench near the pond at the cemetery. With all the constant roller coaster rides of emotions that were happening in my life, I had to think of something light and good.

It was about Christmas, and the thought of celebrating was not in the wind. I was at just about rock bottom, and I could not see the light at the end of the tunnel so to speak. Mark and I were having trouble communicating, mostly because of our depression and the amount of doctor visits and too high expectations on both our parts. He was looking at the fact that his family was in New Jersey and he was stuck in a hospital bed in Connecticut. My family was in RI and would be doing their own thing this Christmas, and I did not see how we could celebrate.

I mentioned my depression to his Mom one day, and she said it was so sad that he could not attend Thanksgiving with them. She was more quiet than usual, and I could see she was upset about our situation and depression. I told her we would be fine and wished her a great Christmas. I had sent over some homemade potato salad that my mom used to make that had pineapple and grapes in it for Thanksgiving and heard they loved it.

Four days before Christmas I got a knock on the door. It was a friend of Mark's who was holding a small tree with lights and ornaments on it. I was so surprised and thought to myself that it was nice but did not see where we were going to have much under it. He stayed for a while and we had some good laughs, which did bring up our spirits.

The following day, we got another knock on the door. When I opened it there were about 10 people standing there singing carols and wishing us a Merry Christmas. Mark could not hear them so I went up to his room and asked him if they could come up and sing. I could see the trepidation in his eyes, but he said yes. They came up and sang some carols, and we talked. It turned out that several of them had relatives who were HIV positive, and one of them was HIV positive. That seemed to make it ok for Mark. We took their numbers, and they went on their way.

Even though I could see the goodwill that was coming my way I had a hard time receiving it well. It was like I was a hypocrite in some way. I was depressed, and nothing could change that. Two days before Christmas, We received two cards in the mail, one from his mom and one from a friend. Both of them were beautiful Hallmark cards and the words in them were so powerful, but it was the words of his mom that blew me away. They made so much sense and coming from the mother of the person we were both losing made the connection so strong. It was this card, the words of the poet and his mom's thoughts and sentiments that changed my life in ways I did not expect or was prepared for.

What right did I have wallowing in my depression and feeling sorry for myself when there were so many in the community who did not have the support we did, or the stamina to continue to heal the best we knew how? I found it amazing how powerful these cards and gestures were. Now remember there was no internet like we have today, and cards were the main form of communication besides the phone, which was attached to the wall in most cases. I believe this is the reason I started sending so many cards out to people who never expected to receive something in the mail. Such a lost tradition.

When I hear horror stories that are happening all around me about the tugging and pulling of emotions and material things, I thank God that the people around Mark and I turned out the way they did. In this world of judgment and sentencing people to whatever fate in the social arena others feel they belong in, it is nice to know there is a light that shines sometimes. That light is love and caring, and a peaceful letting go of a young life, which at times can be so misunderstood.

By the time I got to the house from the cemetery, I must have experienced every emotion possible. The events of the day at the "picnic" gave me another chance to heal and explore my expectations on a real level. I never knew how disorienting an event like the loss of a loved one could be and how things seem to unfold right before my eyes. I felt like I was and still am on an adventure and every corner I turn opens new opportunities and challenges.

Thanks to all of you who were there at his side, my side and his family's side when we needed it. You were all there to the end, even if only in thoughts and prayers. I now know the true meaning of angels on earth.

Thank you.

THE LETTER

A friend of mine messaged me to let me know that he is in remission from cancer. He stated that part of the success of his recovery was due to a letter I sent him a long time ago and he took it to heart. He has asked me to share it so others could read it and think about using it. He was so thankful that I shared it with him. I also just shared it with a school mate who is going through a tough time. I have had nothing but thanks since. So here it goes, and even though I don't want to divulge his or her name for privacy reasons, just think of them as my friends and wish them well.

A manual for surviving a moment in time that one may deem impossible.

Laugh.
Laugh at anything.
Laugh at everything.
Laugh at the way you feel.

Find something funny or at least amusing and wonderful about every part of your body that may have been affected. Imagine you are out of your body and have just met yourself as someone else and see what you see. Be kind to yourself and do not take things too seriously. Make faces in the mirror. You already know what you do not like about yourself now, so find out what you like about yourself and make a list. I have found that sometimes when we make a list, just the act of making a list will lighten the load a bit or can make things more real.

There will be times when you will find yourself in moments that make no sense. Sadness, anger, confusion, frustration and just plain old disgust and depression may appear in moments when you least expect it. Embrace them as your new friend, housemate or companion as you will be living with them for a while. Make up nicknames for them. Make them silly. If you can draw, make them look funny. You already know their ugly head as it has reared up so unjustly.

Forgive it.
It is not you.
It is not who you are.
It is what happened to you.

If you fell would you only be defined as a fall or a person that falls? Yes, some people will define you with nicknames that are unfair. You are more than that.

Ask people to tell you a good joke and allow them to tell one about your ailment. When I cut my finger off and was in the ER, people were so serious and depressing. I asked them to tell me some good finger jokes or jokes about lost fingers. It took a while, but we ended up infecting the whole ER with laughter and smiles which helped me get through it. If you question this, watch the movie Patch Adams.

Now take things seriously and create a logical balance of concern, growth-exploration and sadness, allowing yourself to cry and be sad, allow others to be sad and comfort them when they are and let them know that it is OK. Pity can be your worst enemy. Allow yourself to be sad in the mirror and allow yourself to cry. Cry hard and feel the pain. It will help you later when others are crying and will remind you of the pain. You will not become insensitive to it, but you will be comfortable with it as it is now a new norm you have explored.

Talk to your friends and ask them how they are and how they feel about it. Ask them to be honest about it without fear of hurting you. They must be free from the chains of fear of making a mistake. You want friends who are honest and whole. To find, they have to be willing to express themselves freely. Do this only after you have experienced the most painful moments of sadness and anger by yourself.

Look at this experience of who you are and what has happened to you as a new, beautiful moment with new things to be learned. Write or record your feelings and thoughts, no matter how bad or painful they are. I found that when I wrote, especially poems, I was leaving the pain and concern on the paper as I am now and this, in turn, lightened my load.

Picture yourself in a movie and find a message that you can leave for the world to receive. But just "be" and just write. Ann Frank did not plan on creating a book or message that would spark such a compassionate response to what was happening to people then. The person who wrote "Desiderata" which begins with "Go placidly amid the noise and haste and remember what peace there is in silence" did not know how many people would be profoundly affected by it but this person still wrote it. When I was going through all my pain and concern for what people would think of me, I had a framed copy of Desiderata on my wall which I wake up to every morning.

I was working as a Caregiver for a boy with CP for 20+ years, and when these tragic things happened to me, he guided me through and showed me that life is good no matter how bad it looks. Completely reliant on my moving him, feeding him, changing him and just everyday feelings, he was my joy. He was the one who made me laugh at life, and he was the one who accepted me with one less finger or half of my body not working the way I wanted it to. If I fell, he laughed his ass off. If I stuttered, he made me feel like it was normal and he could understand. He also taught me to get mad when I was mad and get angry when I was angry. He also taught me that after the anger, normalcy can be a welcome friend even if it is not the normal you dream of.

Look for people in your life who can or do lift you. Share a glass of wine with a friend and toast life even if you cannot hold the glass. I have learned that life is a complex box of puzzle pieces with some pieces missing or at least not found. Yet the problem with puzzles is that when you are done and you have completed them, they get put on the shelf for eternity, thrown out or end up at the Thrift Toy section for someone else to figure out. So, do not be upset if your pieces do not all fit together. And if you can, let a friend help you find some pieces.

You will meet a lot of people, and you will know who the people are who have your best interest at heart. Yet there are so many out there that are one step away from that level of caring but cannot find the courage or the knowledge as to how to get there.

Do not judge them too harshly as they could be the ones that will come through someday. I have many students who looked at me as just another adult who worked in the educational system only to find out that I had their backs, no matter how many drugs they take or things they stole. Today some of them are my greatest defenders and allies.

Above all do not give up. One of my strongest moments was when I listened to some music or lyrics of a song that made me cry or inspired me. In this light, Peter Gabriel's "Don't Give Up" played a major role in my recovery and just keeping my sanity.

There were times when I thought I was the only one going through the things I was going through until I googled the word "INSPIRE". I looked at video after video and read excerpt after excerpt of inspiring stories and books about people who have overcome things I could never imagine. That was when I could say I am WHOLE. I am ME. I am OK. I realized that what I was going through, thousands of people have gone through before me, and in many cases in more horrible situations. I was blessed. I was living a charmed and yes at times perverse life with emotions and feelings I was not ready for. But I was OK.

There are times, after a conversation, I will get reactions from people who feel they have gone through worse, and many probably have, like, "Well you were not close to death." I do not know that. "You never had Cancer." I know that. I never wanted this to become a competition or pissing contest. Yet, what I also know is that if I ever do get cancer or a death sentence from an illness, I would like to believe, I will be ready for it. I will be ready, partly from what I went through, or suffered through in self-pity. Much of this readiness is from my experience of sitting at the deathbed of kids who were homeless, on drugs with AIDS and outcasts in our "humane" community. Then there was the boy with CP who was and is as helpless as they come relying on the compassion of everyone and from caring for so many people daily who were just waiting for death to show its face, this is where courage and stamina would come from.

They taught me that there are two miracles that we do not quite understand and may always be a mystery to us. Birth and Death. We can pretend to know or understand where we come from or where we go and I am not saying there is nothing out there as I do believe there is something, but I have had to realize that there is a difference between knowing and believing. I am OK with that and what anyone else knows or believes as it is fuel for conversation.

But life is now. Life is as we know it in our reality. How we translate our now and our reality to allow us to create a livable, sustainable and comfortable experience is up to each one of us individually. We have examples of this throughout history and in our imagination, as we can see in movies, books, and our creativity. It has been said that if you can imagine it, you can be it. I believe that to be true in some experiences and know it to be true in many other experiences.

If you are still one of those who want to wallow in your self-pity and believe I have ruined it for you, or you are mad at me for making it harder to deal with, so be it. That is you and what your reality is now. Just know that you can change whatever you want to change at any time. It may not be comfortable or easy, but it is all about choice and the belief that you have that ability where you are in that reality and whether it is changeable, or not.

I do like to wallow in my pity every so often, and I think it is because I want to remind myself of what that is. I have to admit, sometimes it does feel good.

So, do go placidly. Cry when you can. Get freaking angry. Laugh at yourself. Let your friends be who they are, afraid, concerned and brave enough sometimes to help you pull through this shit. But most of all, live your reality to the fullest.

Do not worry about what others will think, because that will bring you down. Breathe well and often and if you are spiritual, whatever your belief system may be, experience that joy. We are only on this good earth once or are we?

May you live in peace and if you ever think of me, let me know. I have not been able to read minds the way mom did.

So now that I have jumbled the brain cells a bit more, to sum it up, LAUGH. That is all you have to do. The rest will follow.

There is a line in the movie "Fiddler on The Roof" where Papa is talking about his daughter who got married. He said "They are so happy, they do not know how miserable they are."

Lovingly,
Eli

TIME OUT FOR ME...

Looking back at all the commotion during the time I was taking care of Mark, I found it beneficial to take time out for me. By that I mean, being by myself and doing things that I need to do for me, such as relaxing and working on projects. Lately I have been looking at the idea of taking time out for me, as problematic and difficult as it was over 20 years ago, but now I have that history to refer to.

I found it necessary to talk to Mark about it and get his approval and understanding. I also had to let him know I was not going to abandon him in any way but that I just need time to breathe, think and collect my thoughts or just change the scenery. It was not easy, as he came up with the statement "What about my scenery?" I also tended to forget time and talk to people longer than I "should."

At times, I found that the time I had to myself was when he was asleep, at 2:00 A.M. and there wasn't much going on to take my attention away from the issues at hand. TV programs were usually infomercials and old movies, with much fewer channels to surf than we have today. I began making dinners that I could freeze for later to save time, or working on a project I wanted to finish. There was no one to talk to, so it was my time and mine alone. You also have to understand that the computer was still in its early stages.

I began writing, sorting photographs, organizing bookshelves and even developing photos in the darkroom in the wee hours of the morning. I even did a whole photoshoot for Victory Shirt Company who I was working with to develop their catalog, which would come out later that year. I don't think Mark ever got a chance to see it. This was the company Mark had originally worked for and got me involved with in 1984. The original owner, Mary Sprague, was one of the first woman who owned a male oriented business in midtown Manhattan. She had sold it to an employee, and I was part of the deal as I did all the displays, photography and store design by that time. I stayed with the company until 2001 when it closed. The hour of the day did not matter anymore. It was the quality of what I did with that time that mattered. I needed to do something that would make me feel like I was doing something constructive.

After 20+ years, I still have a problem working 9 to 5 but it was the many odd hours I worked that I feel I lost my job recently even though they said it was from budget cuts. I have always had two jobs since I can remember and a multitude of projects. I find that the late hours of the night and early hours of the morning seem to be when I do most of my constructive and creative thinking, as it is now 1:30 A.M. and usually feel like I have accomplished something. My priorities are different, the subject matter may change, but the technique is still the same. No distractions from phones or everyday commitments to take me away from the task at hand.

I am sure we all do this from time to time, looking for that time of day where it is all our own. That was so important to my survival during Mark's and Burt's illness and to the success of my helping them as a Caregiver. It helped because I needed to keep a check on my sense of self when it was so easy to lose it.

Mark and Burt seemed to understand. The nights when I needed my sleep, they would hold in their pain and agony, for the most part, to allow me to gain my strength. Catching up on my rest so I could function later was not always as successful as I had wanted. The body has many ways of telling us that things are not working. In talking to many who have cared for other people with HIV and cancer, that understanding was not as present as it was for me. When someone is in pain, sometimes that is all they can focus on, and it seems like nothing else in the world matters. In Mark's case and in many instances with Burt, they both knew they were also Caregivers.

I think we all can get a glimpse of that when we have a massive headache or a bad case of the flu, and we don't much care about what is happening around us except getting better. We can become very selfish, especially when we are grieving. We may say "Others don't understand," and many times they don't understand, but if we can try to understand where we are in relationship to the reality at hand, we might cope better with the whole picture.

This was something Mark was aware of. He knew if he allowed me to regroup, the next moments or days would be better for him also. Both he and Burt were such giving people in this way, even when they were in their most painful stages. We all understood. That is why we survived each day so well. I remember when I was very young, my parents taught my siblings and I to be aware of where we were when we were not at our best. Whether it was when we were sick, struggling with homework or playing a game that we didn't want to play and we were with friends, and peer pressure came into play we had to be conscious of this. Many times we did not listen, but I have to thank my parents for giving me that sense of self so early on. I am still a bit of a daydreamer at times, but I usually know where I am concerning the reality around me.

After Mark died in 1992 and Burt in 2012, I found myself with a lot of time on my hands. It was that feeling you get when you are going full speed and then stop abruptly. As I have said, the silence is deafening.

What I didn't know at that point, was that I was also the one who was ill. I had a thing called grief, loneliness, depression and boredom. I also had a feeling that I did not know what to do with myself and when I did something, I questioned it. It is an area that many people do not understand, yet they think they know how to help you get over it quicker. I call it The Magic Pill.

People need to grieve in their own time and on their terms. No one should tell another person how that person should grieve or should they? I believe it is fine to tell others how I got through the grieving process, but to instruct others how they need to grieve is wrong. Using the preface "I have heard" can always be a remedy for that. Oh, it's nice to see how others got through it, and it sometimes gives us something to go on or compare to, but the grief must be our own and no one else's, and we must own it on our terms.

Immediately after my losses, I found people calling me and trying to assist me in my grief, but not willing to listen to my grief or acknowledge that it was my grief. Don't get me wrong, there were many who let me grieve my way, with no judgment. Those were the friends I appreciated the most who would say, "If you need anything, just call mem" and gave me the space to grieve and call them when *I felt the need*. That was so important. Grieving is genuinely a solitary and personal event, and when others impose their rules on someone, it can feel like a violation of one's soul. Of course, some show off their grief on their sleeve like a badge of honor. But most of the time, I find that is the result of a very lonely grieving person who needs attention.

I was confronted by many who insisted on taking me out to meet people or to just go out to dinner when all I needed was to be alone and cry or yell or just be quiet by myself. It was so personal at times that we tended to lash out at our best friends and sometimes lost them in the process because they just didn't understand. Yet there are those who I wished I had lost or had gone away but clung like leeches no matter how much I yelled or insulted them. A few who tried so hard and could not see past their own needs probably will never see the damage done. They just did not get that I could not see them in my circle of close friends again. Maybe at some later date, I might have a change of heart. Unfortunately, the more they tried to patch things up, the further away from them I felt. It sounds mean, especially to them, but I have the right to let into my circle of friends who I want to in my life and allow them to share my space. People who are in recovery or rehab can relate to this. Some of the kids I had in school who got into the drug scene and came out of rehab have told me how true this is.

Trust became an issue with me. It became harder and harder to trust people. It was tough letting people into my life which caused the depression I was facing and even affected my job in many ways. Not only was I grieving the loss of my father, Mark, Elsie and later Burt, but the loss of my identity, who I was and who I wanted to be. I was suddenly not the Caregiver anymore, I was the griever. It took a long time to create the me I am. When I found that I was recreating myself, I felt vulnerable. What I also learned was that this vulnerability was like an open the door to better things. I was looking at new opportunities in a different light. Grief changes people and their perspective. But I found that it was easier for people to take advantage of me financially. I was more open to helping others which led to being taken for a ride or advantage of. For the most part, people didn't take advantage in a bad way. Most paid me back if it was money, and if it was helping others I was thanked and paid back later with favors.

I did find that in a time of loss, the vulnerability sets in and becomes tougher than the illness which created the loss. It can become an open door for people looking for love, financial help, friendship when no one else will bite, pity and a host of other opportunistic situations that will begin to surface. I found that when I, and others I have spoken to, are in a state of shock, grief, confusion, loneliness, and fear, it becomes open season for abusers.

Again, the biggest problem came when I just needed to be left alone, and others insisted on jumping in the ring without permission. I would say, "I don't want to talk to you about this right now and don't take offense or take it personally," or "I don't want to be around anyone right now," and they would feel offended or left out, and persist in making appearances. I found myself guilty of this when a former student survived an accident. He was there for me when I needed someone, and I wanted to repay him and be there as often as I could until his mom said, "Enough." It was a bit uncomfortable and felt like I was being pushed away by his mom when all I wanted to do was help as much as I could, but I had to understand that when it was me, I was the one who needed the space to recreate without being recreated. I had to respect his mom's wishes as much as it did hurt my pride.

It has been a hard lesson for me, but I hope I never again fall into a situation where I only listen to my needs when dealing with someone who is going through this grieving process. We all grieve differently because we are all individuals and have diverse backgrounds, cultures and life experiences that have molded us into who we are now. No one can or should dare to recreate someone who has gone through a loss of any sort. Reflecting on what you may have gone through as your experience instead of laying it on others is a better route to take.

I have spent a lot of time trying to understand loss and have found that in allowing others to orchestrate my grief and recovery I was not allowing myself to grieve or heal the way I needed to. These experiences are extremely personal and can affect emotional well being which can prolong the healing process. People have spent millions of hours in the psychiatrist's office all because they weren't allowed or did not have the tools to grieve on their own or they didn't allow themselves to experience their grief. I am not saying that psychiatrists are not a good tool, but sometimes I think society does not allow any other way.

Time out is needed in everyday life and especially after loss whether it be a loved one, a pet, a job, a material item or a spiritual loss. When we come to that level of consciousness that we can allow ourselves and others the time needed, we all gain from that action and our inner wisdom.

Mark's ability to allow me time out and Burt's ability to let me sleep unconditionally, when they were capable of doing so, came about gradually but made us stronger and more patient with each other. It was a lesson I hope to never forget and one I hope I can share with others when the time arises. If we don't take control of who we are and who or what we allow in our lives, we lose control. Sure, we may close some doors at times and lose out on opportunities, but I found that it has that control that makes all the difference.

So, take time out and take control. It isn't easy at times when all fingers seem to be pointing at you in blame, accusation and judgment when you may be at your most vulnerable. But doing it can bring you to a higher sense of self as it did for me. It all boils down to you being you.

The feelings we all have are so individual and unique for each of us. The strength that will help us succeed in our grief comes from letting us feel the feelings. Grief is an emotion and to ignore it will postpone its success. Grief like many things has a life of its own in so many ways. For each person, the direction it takes will be different. To compare it with another person's experience is unfair. The more you deal with your grief, the less you will see intrusive moments in your life. Many times, I felt guilty of not grieving the way I thought I should have, and I felt like I shortchanged the person I lost. This is a natural response, but not to worry. It does get better and easier even if it does not go away. I am sure you have heard that before.

SUPPORT FROM A HIGHER SOURCE...

It was Mother's Day only a few months after moving to Connecticut. I found myself in need of paying respects to my mother, who had died ten years before. Guilt may have had something to do with it but the need to do this was there. I had heard of a church in Stamford, St John's Episcopal, and being raised Episcopalian, I had to go in and say a few prayers.

Not being much of a church-going person at the time, (although I do feel I am a very spiritual soul) and given that I entered with hesitation, I sat in the back pew closest to the door, probably preparing myself for an easy exit. The church was huge and architecturally quite glorious with its tall stained-glass windows and towering arched nave made of carved stone. Quite imposing yet quite welcoming in its own glorious way. I have always had an interest in studying stained glass, and as a photographer I was doubly interested, as they made wonderful subjects to photograph and the natural light made it an easy subject technically.

This imposing structure was distracting enough that I forgot why I was there, but only for a bit. During the sermon, I heard the minister in the pulpit saying things about motherhood and using some stories in the bible, which had one of the most amazing mother stories ever, to validate his sermon. His name I would later find out was Leander Harding and he had an amazing way about him and with his parish. In time, I would find him to be one of my greatest supporters during the loss of my dad, and Mark's illness and eventual death.

During his sermon, he said some things that spiked my senses. What they were I don't recall, but over time, they helped me feel free from the chain I had allowed to weigh me down with guilt about not being complete with my mother. His soft and kind voice drew me into the service and made me feel at home. He was doing his job and doing it well.

My mother's death was sudden. She had experienced a heart attack and stroke and went into a coma for a brief time. Unfortunately, it was not long enough for me to see her while she was in the hospital. I had been working in Andover, Mass at a group home for adults with disabilities, which was an amazing job. These young adults would prove to be one of my most valuable support systems during this time. Even though my mom and I spoke to each other on an almost daily basis, I felt there were many things unsaid. I am told that this often happens to people who lose their loved ones from sudden death. It seems we never say things we want to say or "should" say while they are alive. This tends to leave a gap in our lives leading to a feeling of guilt and accompanied by an extended sense of loss added to the physical loss of a loved one.

While I was working in Andover at the group home, I received a call from my sister telling me that Mom had gone to the hospital after suffering a heart attack and stroke. She told me about the coma, and she was holding on, but I should think about getting down there. I had just spoken to Mom the night before, and she sounded fine, so I thought I would have some time to get someone to take my shift and talk to the residents about what had happened.

The next day I sat down with all the residents and told them the situation. Several of them had lost a parent, so they were not unfamiliar with the loss of a family member. One of the residents came up to me and sat with me to console me. She had lost a parent and several other family members, and in her own way, she was telling me it would be ok. It was so sweet how they looked after me in this time of uncertainty. I found someone to take my shifts and the next day I took a bus to Boston to connect with the train to Providence. When I got to the train station, I called my brother-in-law who was to pick me up at the Providence station.

The phone call went a little like this.

> Me: "Hi Duke. I am at the Boston station. I will be in Providence in about an hour. How is Mom doing?'
>
> Duke: "You didn't hear?"
>
> Me: "No, how is she?"
>
> Duke: "She passed away about an hour ago, and the family is here."
>
> Me: "I know but, how is she?"
>
> Duke: "Just get down here as soon as you can."
>
> Me: "OK see you later."

The train was about to leave, and I had to run to catch it, so my mind was not clear. I got on and found a seat, got some reading material out and we started to roll. As it started moving at a good clip, I started to think about my conversation with Duke. Suddenly I realized he had told me she had passed away, which hit me as if I had run into a brick wall. There I was in a train car, all alone with a lot of strangers, tears running down my cheeks and not knowing what to do. I have never felt so alone.

I began to think about all the conversations I had recently with my mom hoping I was "complete" with her. I felt so guilty about not saying "I love you" several times and a few arguments we had. Not a good feeling to have.

I carried that with me for more than ten years till that Mother's Day at St John's in Connecticut. Listening to Leander's sermon would help me be complete with my mother and eventually help me with my father's death and even more so, with Mark's death. I felt better about my spiritual relationship with my mom that day after so many years feeling I didn't have one.

After every late Sunday service, the church had a coffee hour where parishioners could mingle and relax with each other. I wanted to tell Leander how much his sermon helped me and felt this would be an opportune time to do that. As with most coffee hours, you have the recruiters who were out in force. Being the artful dodger that I was, I quickly grabbed my coffee and headed for Leander. I thought being with him might keep me from the claws of the recruiters. No such luck. He was the head recruiter and a good one at that. I was hooked.

During our conversation, I got a chance to thank him for his sermon and tell him how much I got out of it and how much it transformed my sense of being complete with mom. He was quite impressed that I had listened so closely and thanked me for the compliments.

I didn't share that experience with anyone for a long time. It was as if it was between me, my mom and Leander. This encounter later gave me the courage to speak to him and no one else about what I was going through as Mark's Caregiver. It seemed all I needed was for him to listen to me, and he was a professional listener indeed. This listening, I believe, is so important to Caregivers during the time they are giving care and it is as important as it is for the people being cared for to be listened to about what they are going through. His responses were always reassuring, and I always walked out of his office feeling like a weight had been lifted. I sometimes feel that just the act of talking is what lifted the weight. He also helped me feel like I wasn't alone in all this.

During the beginning of Mark's illness, Leander was the only person with whom I could share my pain. There was so much judgment surrounding me elsewhere just because I was associated with someone who was HIV positive that I was only able to open up to a select few of my closest friends, and even then I was hesitant.

I remember one day I had gotten to the end of my rope. I was exhausted, frustrated and confused. I had just spent the night helping Mark with his swollen feet by massaging them as he was losing sensation in them at a fast pace. He wanted his coffee the first thing that morning, and I forgot to get a can of coffee the day before, so we had none left.

In his frustration, he began to yell, and the anger caused him to say things I knew he didn't mean. I was hurt and left the apartment at about 9:00 AM to do some jobs but felt I needed to talk to someone as soon as possible. I remembered Leander, and the first few times I spoke to him. Even though by now I was a member of the congregation, I had not sat in council with him for some time. I felt it was time again. I stopped by the church office hoping he would be there and have some time for me. I walked in and spoke to the secretary. The sun was reflecting off the windows of the buildings across the lawn, which made the room seem magical as the windows in her office were colored glass and leaded glass.

"Hi," I said hesitantly, "is Father Harding in?"

"Yes," she said, "Do you have an appointment with him...." As her voice faded. I think she saw I needed to talk to someone. "Wait here. I will see if he is free."

My nerves and patience were wearing on me, and the short time she was gone seemed a lot longer. She came back and said, "Go right in." Those were three of the nicest words I had heard all day.

As I walked up to the door, which was open a crack, I could see his figure sitting at the desk writing. Flashbacks of going to the principal's office crossed my mind. My first thought was that he was too busy and I should not interrupt him. I began to think of ways to excuse myself, but I knocked, and he opened the door. "Come in, Eli." he said, "It is good to see you. What can I do for you?" I didn't know where to begin so I just started talking, and I am sure at times it seemed like I was babbling. I told him about Mark's condition and my condition at this point and did not know where to go from here. I couldn't talk about the subject without tears, and holding them back made it even harder.

He listened, asked a few questions and said, "There isn't much I can do, as you are doing as much as you can already. Coming to talk about it was the right thing to do. I could refer you to some groups if you feel ready or counseling, if you feel you need it. What I will offer you is this office any time you feel the need to talk with someone. Sometimes all we need is a good listener." That, I was aware of.

Getting it out and knowing it wouldn't go any further, sort of a safe zone, was important, which I am sure you understand if you are any kind of Caregiver. Sometimes I found myself being my own judge and jury. It was nice getting a second opinion, so to speak.

He then said, "Let us pray."

I wish I could remember the prayer he said. I remember it had an impact on how I felt and where I was going. I really think it gave me some strength to continue with caring for Mark, even after just losing my father.

One of the biggest problems I found with caregiving, for me anyway, was that we feel there is a need to talk to someone and many times we don't or can't find the right person or safe zone. This is not just true for Caregivers, but also for people being cared for as I recently found while helping Brian, the former student, now friend, who I mentioned earlier in the book and had suffered a TBI from a car accident. He was thrown from his car, hitting a stone wall. His recovery and self-care have given me a glimpse of how hard it is not to be able to confide in others safely. We talk a lot even now after 6 years. It is like we hold back for fear of exposure, anxiety, being judged and the knowledge that society can be unintentionally cruel. It reminds me of when I was a kid and I was afraid the others would laugh if I did something stupid or did not meet their standards or fit in. But now I am in the adult world, and this still holds true. We all judge and are judged.

At times, I feel that society puts too much emphasis on the causes and reasons why, and not enough on the problem at hand. By this I mean, some feel that if someone is HIV positive, they are stupid or careless or are this or that, instead of just acknowledging the fact that they are HIV positive and no other judgment. We do this all through society. My son is African American. He has opened my eyes wide to the judgments and persecutions we subconsciously put on others because they are a different color, religion, culture, gender, or social status. To this day, we are still doing this and to be honest, I believe that it will not change any time soon. That is who we are. We are different colors, religions, cultures, genders and social statuses, and if it is us and them we see first, we will always place judgments to survive. There are so many people out there suffering in silence. Groups like the support groups that I have attended, churches and safe zones are making a difference. Yet it is still up to the individual to make that step to get help or support.

Many Caregivers are too busy giving care and don't see this need until it is too late. They feel alone, like they are the only ones who are going through this. I don't have enough fingers and toes to count the times I felt like this. We say, "Who would understand anyway?" I believe it is OK to ask for help if you feel comfortable with where you are getting it from. We sometimes label things important only when they affect us directly as in a crisis. The death toll from a disaster like an earthquake or a hurricane or a fire or AIDS is a tragedy. Its importance is many times determined by how close we are to it. When people go through disasters, it is hard to understand why everyone else isn't there to help or they don't think it is important.

In 2011, Hurricane Irene hit the area in Vermont where I have been living for the past 20 years. Communities were completely cut off from the rest of the world. Many people could not understand Vermont having floods, as we were in the Green Mountain Range. So how could we have flooded? Cut off like that, people who were not directly affected and could not feel the urgency of Hurricane Katrina in the south were now living the anger and frustration and urgency of what comes with disasters like this. It took 6 months of reconstruction and good neighbors to finally realize how urgent it was. Then there was the hurricane that hit Puerto Rico and the politics that went on while people who were and still are cut off from the world cannot understand why no one cares. I am sure if we all were hit the same way, we would have a different perspective. It is the same for Caregivers and people being cared for, where the urgency of getting support and help is not felt by the general population as they go about their daily lives. I am just as guilty of this as anyone and will be again. But if I am aware of it, I can do something about it; freedom of choice also needs knowledge and awareness.

Asking for help is the first and biggest step in becoming a healthy Caregiver. I am glad I dared to take that step and am prepared to again. One of the questions in a book I am working on is, "Where do you think courage comes from?" It took a long time for me to see this. I feel it comes from my experience in life and is connected to my comfort zone, as well as to everyone I have met. But most of all it comes from something inside called survival and love. This is where the fear comes from, so be prepared to juggle. That is why knowledge of the situation or illness, and awareness of who you are and what you are doing, is so important.

If I were purposely going to jump off a cliff, my courage to do it would be determined by whether I had jumped off anything taller than myself, who my teacher was, what I was going to land on, whether there was imminent danger coming my way and how big the cliff was. If it meant the difference between life or death, that is one thing. If it meant overcoming the fear of trust in someone or something, it would become more complicated and difficult.

Taking the chance to trust someone with your pain and hoping to gain strength from that trust is what Caregivers must deal with. I am sure it is true for victims of cancer, AIDS or any situation that pulls your emotional strings and sense of survival. If the person you are caring for dies, it gets even harder. Most of us sweep our feelings of pain and confusion under the rug and try to go on with our lives. I tried to do that in the beginning and thought I was the strong one, but the rug got so bumpy from all the things I was sweeping under it and was hard to walk over it and balance myself, which means that I had a lot of baggage I was not dealing with. It also ends up causing more confusion and pain. At least it did for me. We are all different.

The help we need can come from many different places, people, pets, books, music, food, etc. One has to feel comfortable with the source of the help and has to receive it in one's own time. It means giving someone the space to accept help. We then must try not to bombard that person with too much help at one time.

The day Mark died, I felt like I had been driving for thousands of miles and all of a sudden, the car stopped. The deafening quiet, the feeling of loss and not knowing what to do next, was overwhelming. The termination of all the activities such as caring, hoping, feeding, cooking for him, cleaning, shopping, washing bed sheets, setting up appointments and putting my life on hold for someone I cared so much about and loved so much was devastating, to say the least. When it all came to a halt, I had to pick up the pieces and try to go on. Not an easy thing to do, especially if you haven't had that experience before in life.

Reading all the books and listening to all the talk shows and programs on the subject sometimes is not enough. It takes work, support, and determination to get to a calmer place in time. Sometimes even from a higher power.

We all carry what I call our little bag of "shoulda/coulda/woulda" seeds and are more than willing to spread them around. We also put ourselves through the "shoulda/coulda/woulda" phase almost willingly. I should have done this, or I could have done it this way, or I would have been better at it if… Then comes the "if only" group. If only I had done it this way or said this different. I found myself doing this to justify who I was and where I was at any given moment. I became my own judge, jury, and worst enemy.

I found that writing could be a tool in working my way through the thickets in this briar-filled garden we call caregiving, which is just a small piece of the larger garden called life. It gave me a chance to talk to myself and not get caught doing it. Looking back at my notes, I came up with some wild analogies. Each of us has to find our own path and hope that it will take us to where we want to be. I have come to believe that my biggest support was from a Higher Source.

Thanks, Mom.

P.S. When I did get back that day Mark got mad, we had an amazing talk and got the chance to tell each other what we felt. It's all good.

SPIRITUALITY

For many years, I was under the belief that spirituality and religion were the same. This might be true for a lot of us. I know now that they are separate pieces of the whole pie, even though they intertwine in our lives quite often.

The definition of spiritual reads,

1. "The spirit of the soul as distinguished from the body or material matters."
2. "From or concerned with the intellect; Intellectual."
3. "Showing much refinement of thought and feeling."

These can be related to religion and the religious components of our societies. To be a spiritual person, one needs to feel, have some level of self-esteem, be a part of something or someone, (as in a relationship), fit in somewhere in the social structure and open the mind to new things, feelings and deeds. I have come to believe that we as social beings need to be connected somewhere to get feedback and have a sense that we belong to something bigger than us. Granted, spirituality can come in many more forms than just discussed, and some subscribe to the belief that spiritualists need no other support. I found that when some of these other components are in line, it creates more room for constructive and clutter-free spirituality.

Climbing this caregiving mountain as a self-proclaimed Caregiver, I found myself looking for a foothold in all the challenges I had to meet to get to where I needed to be at one time or another. While Mark was living with HIV, I could see him searching and trying to fit in somewhere that would validate his situation. Yet when he became even sicker and had full-blown AIDS as he called it, I could see him trying to find something to fill a series of empty places. It is hard to explain unless you have ever felt like you did not belong. If you did belong, the empty spaces would be filled with other positive elements in your life. If you did not belong or felt left out in some way, the struggle to fit in will have become all-consuming, and it presents a lot of questions and unknowns.

Because Mark and I were so close, I found it hard filling his empty spaces when I had some of them also. By empty space, I mean somewhere in your heart or spirit you don't feel complete. It could mean not doing or not being able to do something you always wanted to do or not saying something to someone you felt the need to say or just being in a frame of mind that can stall you like you just pressed the hold button. When you call some office or agency, and they put you on hold, you generally sit there listening to the most horrible music for as long as they wish to keep you waiting. The feeling of being insignificant prevails. It is like that.

I didn't quite understand spirituality until I found myself not feeling sorry for him, but feeling the sorrow. To me, feeling sorry is a facade covering the surface. The word "sorry" in our culture has connotations of "I can't help" or "I am not willing to go any deeper into the matter." We seem to use the phrase "I'm sorry" too freely and it does not mean anything other than "I said it so now forgive me." Have you ever heard anyone say "Sorry doesn't cut it"?

There have been many times when I had a lot of change in my pocket, and a homeless person was asking for money. My immediate response was to say "Sorry" and walk away as if I had to protect my assets. Or when I have raised my hand, palm facing toward them and said "Sorry," meaning I can't or won't help. That is feeling sorry.

Feeling the sorrow is a level deeper into our spirituality or soul. Feeling the sorrow allows us to act on it, no excuses, and feel it on a deeper level. As a Caregiver on the family and friend level, it becomes easier to feel the sorrow as we may feel obligated and can better understand and help those we love. On the professional level, it becomes a different animal and is almost taboo to get close enough to feel the sorrow. Nurses must rely on their knowledge and expertise rather than their spirituality, because getting too close and feeling the sorrow could cause burn out. Don't get me wrong; I know many nurses, EMTs, and doctors who are some of the most compassionate people anyone would want to meet, but it takes a lot to get to that point and not burn out. Feeling the sorrow becomes a mechanism of the profession that can go either way. It either could work well or become a disaster. Therefore, it is harder for families and friends to be primary Caregivers than the professionals as it requires the person to go through training. Families usually are thrown into it with no training and rely on the gut and soul to get them through it.

This is where I have seen a deep gap between the family and the professionals, and there will always be a bit of mistrust on both sides. Until we begin to acknowledge that the family needs much more training that is available to them and incorporate it into our medical institutions successfully, family and friends will always be at a loss, and that is where the mistrust, or on the other side of the coin, the blind trust lives. We may sometimes look at the medical profession as cold and mechanical, but in recent times I have seen some real changes and collaborative efforts to work together.

I spoke to some nurses at a hospital about how hard it must be to go through this, day in and day out. They responded that it was all part of the job. It was something that they had to be trained to not let affect them. I guess if it were a part of my job I would feel like them, but families and friends must go to a place much deeper to fill the empty space.

I worked as a Caregiver for a boy with CP for about 20 years, and in those 20 years I worked as a professional, but in many cases, I became like family. I can see the dilemma, and yet I now have a wonderful friend who lives in South Carolina who I call every day, even just to say hi. I can see how it can be tough, but I also can see how the two styles can live together and work well.

As I mentioned in a previous chapter, I looked in the library for information about caregiving. The closest thing I found that could relate close enough to help a primary Caregiver handbook for family and friends was the one suggested to me concerning pet care. Constant unconditional love was a rule of thumb, as well as learning to know the pet's needs and at any given time. Pets, like loved ones, can become dependent on us being able to handle their needs without them telling us. You must remember, there was not that much out there for families who were caring for a loved one in the 80s and 90s, and especially about AIDS which was not talked about widely. Unless you could read between the lines, you were left to your own devices.

Now there is more awareness, and with the internet, you can get answers to almost any question. Facebook even has pages just for Caregivers like the Caregivers Space where people can post and share so much that can help so many. I also suggest that you take it upon yourself to read as much as possible with all the new information out there on caregiving and talk to others who have gone through it, which to me was my salvation. I am sure there are some good outlets and these days hospitals have a lot more to offer. What I also found was that all Caregivers go through different situations in very different ways. I found there were so many stages or events I had to experience before I felt comfortable feeling the sorrow. I also suggest that you open a good line of communication with the one you are caring for, so that you can better tailor your care to the needs at hand.

After looking at the pet care book and transposing the information and taking some of its suggestions, I thought it very strange that we sometimes care for our pets with more spirituality and love than we do our loved ones. I have seen this in situations where parents have experienced a child getting hurt and ending up with a TBI. In many cases just saying to this person, "you used to do things differently" or "I remember when we used to...". The person may not remember who they were before the accident and it can cause so much more stress and setbacks. This is when feeling the sorrow can go too far. I am not saying that is true for everyone, but I still see it. With the number of books there were on pet care compared to the few books I found to help me care for Mark in the 90s, it made me wonder.

My job in the late 90s was working with the homeless, substance abusers and people with HIV. I have taken many workshops and courses to help me work more effectively with my clients and not lose my "self". One of the workshops about "How We Care" became a very self-revealing experience for me. It had an exercise where we would look at hypothetical situations such as,"If you were walking on the sidewalk and came across a man who was hungry and seemingly helpless and a dog who was hungry and seemingly helpless, which one would you help?".

When I heard this I had a chill down my spine, as I had been in a similar situation once had. I had to admit, I helped the dog and took it to the pound, and there was a seemingly homeless man sitting on some steps. I wonder how many of us would help the man and take him to the doctor or shelter. I know, the man could have had the wherewithal to do it on his own. The dog didn't. In any case, I still feel the guilt.

The second situation was, "If you had come across the same dog, but it was a small child or youth instead of the man?" I began to see my belief system had levels of need, helplessness or priorities that were selective. The levels were determined by how helpless the individual was, whether I felt comfortable with the one I was going to help, as well as whether the person posed a threat. I found out that it also depended on how I felt sorrow or if I felt sorry. The dog and the child got there for distinct reasons and the man "should" be more able to make choices. I became a judge and jury. I also realized that a lot of my reactions were based on my experience with any of these subjects.

Another aspect of this journey was the shame/guilt game. Mark at times would flip-flop between shame and guilt, as would I in certain stages of the illness. For me to be successful in caring for him, I had to better understand the difference between shame and guilt. It took a while, but after reading and listening to some of my friends in the church through sermons and gospel readings, I began to understand how we subconsciously define these two demons, one being easier to work with than the other.

At those times when shame showed its face, Mark would feel like he was a mistake. It became an all-consuming threat to the quality of care he would receive and/or accept. On the other hand, with guilt, it seemed easier because instead of being a mistake, he only made a mistake. He could own only the part of the problem whereas, with shame, he was the whole problem. It can be a hard concept to grasp, but when seen in this light it makes it easier to deal with. If someone makes a mistake, the mistake can be corrected. If someone is a mistake, it is almost impossible to find the correction.

It is hard to move the spirit when shame and guilt get in the way of someone's self-esteem. With the lack of self-esteem, the elements of dignity, pride and at times hope seem far out of reach. At this point I would lose my sense of self, and when I did Mark seemed to follow. Who had we become? We know what we are by what we do, (as in if you teach, you are a teacher), but who we really are becomes a subliminal journey we can't see until we acknowledge some of the results of self-loss, like shame, guilt, and loss of self-esteem. It is like driving in a rainstorm. We know the road is out there, but the rain blurs the vision. We know who we are, but the situation blurs the vision.

One of the things that kept me strong during this whole journey was, a sense of love and belonging or acceptance which, looking back at the definitions, makes sense. Someone on a radio talk show recently asked the question, "Is love a feeling or an action?" I think it is both. There were times when I was so mad at Mark for saying something or for giving me a hard time, one would never know we were close, and I really loved him. But if I didn't have love for him, I wouldn't have made sure his coffee was there each morning without him asking and wouldn't have cleaned and cooked without grumbling when he was mad at me. Love is a feeling, an action and much more.

It was not easy putting my everyday activities on hold so we could get through this journey. I feel lucky that I was able to become the Caregiver I was, even though in the end we didn't know where the next dollar was going to come from. That underlying love for each other made the difference.

Caring for him was truly a spiritual experience, and even though I wish he didn't have to go through it, I wouldn't trade the experience of it for the world. We both grew, and the experience strengthened our spirit. I remember he was so strong for his friends a few days before he died. He received them at the hospital to the point where he couldn't do it anymore. It was so hard for me to tell his best friends that he couldn't see them any longer, no matter how much he wanted to. It was almost like he was getting his spiritual baggage packed for the journey he was about to take.

For many of us, it would be a hard thing to do. I remember talking to someone who was HIV positive and hearing him say "We get all psyched up and ready for the trip to heaven, but when the train is ready to pull out, we freak out." Remembering Mark's last words "Help me, help me, help me," and then silence, makes me think that it is true for all of us at some point. Even though I know he felt ready for it, it still scared him. I know people will say if he was more religious or believed in God (or whatever you believe) more profoundly he would not have been scared. Maybe.

I have to admit, some of the things I have found helpful in raising my spirituality are the simplest things like the quiet of sitting in an empty church, photography, the music of Yanni and Enya, good healthy comedy, laughter, healthy food, exercise, good company and writing this book. I thought that me being a relatively intelligent person and sensitive to many things around me, I could heal myself. Becoming spiritual is its own journey, and it takes a multitude of events, qualities, and experiences to make it work and to find that higher place we all want to attain.

I soon realized I couldn't do it all by myself. I needed to talk to those who have gone through it or at least people who would listen, not judge, and care without smothering me. I also found I had to beware of the "super healers," those people who had all the answers but with hidden agendas. I had several of those who felt I should be well on my way to recovery after a few sessions or meetings with them. These people or groups can delay the recovery or healing process. In some cases, where I took possession of the others' healing processes or mimicking how they healed without knowing it, it began to not look anything like my healing process. I don't think they realized the damage they did in telling me that this was the way to do it with no variations.

I find that healing is a very personal, private and selective process that takes time and patience. There are times even now when I feel I still have a long way to go, and yet other times I feel like I'm there. What I found helpful was listening to others who are healing and are at various stages. I didn't feel alone or crazy after seeing how normal some of the feelings I had were. The difference was, I was listening and not being lectured to.

In 1995 I was part of the founding year of a camp for people infected and affected by HIV/AIDS. I went there as a photographer and counselor for a group of kids whose status was only disclosed by the person if they wished. Otherwise, it was confidential. I didn't know how important this camp would be to how I felt meeting people in my situation or how it would change my life until I began to listen to those who were HIV positive. Outside of camp, there was little acceptance in the community at large and little room for good self-esteem. Mark had passed away three years before I got involved with the camp, and it was still hard to talk about it. There at the camp it was OK to be who you were with what you had or didn't have. It was at this camp where I found that the art of listening was becoming my new best friend. Many times, I tend to appear that I am listening when I am preparing in my mind how I am going to respond. I also met a young man who would later have a profound effect on my life. His name was Homer.

Today, I feel lucky that I was able to meet some incredible people during this journey. There is one thing I feel that is super important as an aid or element of healing: learning how to laugh and see the lighter side of things. I found this in a local support group for people who have lost someone or are in the process of caring for someone. Everyone in this group is either affected or infected or in bereavement. It was like I had someone to walk with who cared, but knew I had to also make it on my own.

We all grasp at straws when we lose something or someone, and knowing that there is someone out there who knows our pain makes it easier or just safer. I worked with clients who were HIV positive every day and still found myself not knowing what to say sometimes or worrying that I may have said or done the wrong thing. It is a fine line to walk. I was dealing with many sensitive people who were looking at the possibility of dying soon. This is normal, and my only answer to this is to do what you feel is right and do it with love. It may hurt sometimes, but if it is done out of love and caring, it will be OK. People can see through that - sometimes not right away but they usually will see it.

I recently called someone who was, as he called it, "desperately depressed and almost suicidal". I said to him, "If there is anything I can do for you, let me know." His response was "There is nothing anyone can do for me."

I took a chance and called him again only to hear a cheerful voice, and a grateful thank you for thinking of him. As I had thought, the drugs and the pain were the cause of his words. If he knew it was the drugs and not him that brought him to this level, he could feel safe. Also, knowing that I didn't forget him or give up on him made a world of difference.

He was trying to go it alone, as was I, and after a while he realized that he needed to talk to a group or a buddy. It seems that when we acknowledge the fact that we need someone else, it is a sign that we are desperate or giving in or giving up. Not true. It is a sign that we are not ready to give up and are ready to go the distance.

This is so true in recovery, healing or attaining wellness. I see people recovering from drug abuse, illness or loss and when they finally reach out to get help, they find out that it is the beginning of the second half. Sometimes I feel we stay at half time too long. But each of us must reach for more _**when we are ready**_.

I don't claim to be an authority on these subjects; I only claimed to have gone through a lot of them and to have climbed the caregiving and healing hill. I hope that by sharing my journey, it will help someone else. We don't always have enough out there for the Caregiver on the layman's level, and the way I look at it is that if we take care of the Caregivers, the people they are caring for will see the difference. It isn't easy sometimes, but we can begin to acknowledge those who care. I can't emphasize enough the saying, "When one gets sick, two or more feel the pain."

Note that this was originally written in 1996. Since then many edits and changes have occurred. 2016 was slated the Year of the Caregiver. A lot has happened, and yet the Caregiver is still struggling. Spirituality has grown to be an integral part of our living in our society. I am blessed to have found mine at a young age, and have honed and developed it throughout the years.

A COLOR SPECTRUM

I grew up in Rhode Island on a street where most of the population was Portuguese, in a village called Clyde. It had the biggest Portuguese American festival, around Labor Day weekend, in a town that was cut up into little ethnic villages. This cultural diversity originated with the mills and mill villages where each ethnic group would gravitate to. The mills, which employed the people from their ethnic background, grew and prospered right up to the late 50s. Artic village was French, Natick was Italian, and Clyde was Portuguese. West Warwick was one of the most ethnically diverse towns in the Northeast, save Boston or NYC. I was so used to hearing languages I did not connect with, and it wasn't until 1970 after coming back from a year in Brazil that I realized that "Via para casa" did not mean "Hi, how are you?" but "Go home." Having that exposure and curiosity about different cultures gave me a solid base for my future endeavors. I remember asking my mom, "If everyone around us speaks Portuguese, why don't we?" She tried to explain that Grandma and Grandpa came from England and they don't speak Portuguese there.

Living and playing with so many people of different cultures opened my eyes and mind about the diversity of the world at a young age. For the most part, I had only been exposed to people who looked and acted relatively the same as me. It was not until I went to the beach with my family that I was exposed to different races. Now I must tell you, this was during the early 50s, and the TV was a new experience. I remember the first TV set we got, which was in about 1953 when I was 5 years old. There were only two channels, Channel 10 and 12, and they were all white. You would never see a black person unless it was on the news. At the age of 5, I was not that interested in world affairs.

While at the beach, I noticed way down the other end of the beach there were some kids who seemed to be having a blast. I wanted so badly to be able to join them as they were playing in the mud and were covered head to toe. It looked like so much fun. When I asked my mom if I could go and join them, she said, "no, it is too far down the beach, and we are all settled on our blankets", plus we were close to the Carousel which I loved. This had happened several times.

It was not until many years later when my mom told me that the reason I gave her was that they were playing in the mud and it looked like fun. At that time, I guess my mom was not sure how to explain it to me that they were not playing in the mud, but that was the color of their skin. It would not be until I was about 10 or 11 that I would meet my first black friends at church camp.

I had heard of them in the children's song in church. The lyrics were, "Jesus loves the little children, all the children of the world, red and yellow, BLACK and white, they are precious in his sight." At that age, they were just words and did not mean much. At camp, in my cabin, there was a kid named Lee who was black as black could be and to be honest, I did not pay it any mind until one of the other kids called him the "N" word. I did not know what that was except what I had heard in the children's rhyme, Eeny Meeny Miny Moe. You may know the rest. Lee and I hit it off and even though I was fascinated by his different skin pigment, it was so easy to foster that friendship, and I think he was just as amazed by how well we got along. As I found out later, he was in a city school that was slowly being integrated, and there was a distinct wall between black and white. We did not have the segregation signs saying white only or black only, but the invisible wall was there.

This was the beginning of my awareness of how society looked at the differences in skin colors. I started hearing whispers about me hanging with the colored kid. I still did not understand until I was told I could not be on a team as we were picking sides for teams. They did not say why but no one picked Lee and me. Luckily the counselor I had insisted that I get picked and I was, for the first time, on the opposing team that Lee was on. I don't remember much about the rest of the week, but I knew that Lee was a good friend.

I never saw Lee again, but it opened my eyes to so much about the fact that he was a decent person and we got along so well. I could not understand the bits and pieces of racist remarks I had heard and that I was called an "N" lover by some. I was not as aware of how differently societies looked at this situation until I became the Assistant Director of a camp like program that was in the basement of the library in Providence RI which was connected to a predominantly black housing project called Chad Brown Projects. I guess I was so ignorant of the dangers of someone like me walking into these projects because I did it many times to talk to some of the parents of the kids who did not come in for a couple of days. The parents were welcoming because they knew who I was, but I am sure they thought I was a nutcase for taking that walk into their world alone. For whatever reason, I didn't feel threatened and I was able to recruit more kids to come to the Library Camp.

When I was in high school in the 60s, the first black family moved into the area and was well accepted by the community and my class. Graduation day came, and when he got his diploma, he got a round of applause for his accomplishments and grade point average. I think he was so well received because it was also who we were as a community of such diverse extremes and who he was as a human being.

In the 1970s I was selected to go to Brazil for a year with the 4-H where, after reading all the material and books on Brazil, I assumed I would be immersed in the black Brazilian culture. My first indication that I would be dead wrong was when I was driven to the Casa de Harmonia Student House. Everyone there was Japanese and spoke both Japanese and Portuguese which challenged me as I had just spent a month learning Portuguese. The time came for me to go to my village where I would meet my Brazilian family who I would be living with for the first month of my stay. The name of the family I was going to live with was Terabe which, to someone who didn't know better, sounded like a Portuguese name.

The bus trip from Sao Paulo was an all-nighter and did not give me any view of the terrain I was going to be living in. The sun began to rise and I started to see people, mostly darker-skinned and living in shacks or huts on the side of the road. By all indications, this was the culture of the people I would be living with for a year. The bus entered the city of Uraí, Paraná, which was typical adobe-looking buildings, a plaza in the center of town and a lot of wooden houses. The bus stopped, and I got off. I knew someone was going to meet me, but I was alone at the stop. Across the street, there was a group of people, a family standing from tallest to smallest. Some had Japanese clothing, but most were dressed in typical Brazilian farm clothing. The oldest man came across the street and bowed in front of me. He then looked at me and said in broken English, "You, Hobert?" which is how Robert, my true first name, is pronounced in Portuguese. "Me Papa." Yes, the family was Japanese. We were all introduced and off we went to the farm I was to live on.

I was filled with a mixture of fear, excitement, and curiosity as I began to settle in. It was getting close to noon, and we all assembled in the kitchen for, what I was to become accustomed to, Café. Café is a break between breakfast and lunch where we would have some coffee, which was very strong and some sweets. I met the rest of the family and got a tour of the property, which was wonderful and full of cactus and bamboo. That evening after supper I wanted to go to bed early, but I had to go to the bathroom which I had not seen in the house. Not knowing much Portuguese, it became a real chore to explain that I had to go to the bathroom. Most of the responses were looks of confusion and amusement. Totally frustrated about not being able to get it across, I took my host brother in the other room and put my hands between my legs and crossed my legs and pleaded, I have to pee. He laughed and said, "OK I know." He took me to the back of the house and pointed down the stairs and in the back yard where there was an outhouse. The sense of relief was euphoric. I think that I was more relieved that I was able to make someone understand me with my limited ability to speak the language.

Outside, it was dark, but I could see the outhouse about 50 feet away. It was hard to understand, but I figured I could maneuver around to figure it out. I took one step forward, and my foot plunged into a sea of muck. Pulling my foot out I lost a shoe. Gone forever. I then went out and around the side and took a pee behind the building. Frustrated, I walked up the stairs and tried to get someone's attention. No one came to the door, so I took one of the bamboo poles leaning up against the back of the house and knocked. My host mom came to the door and began to laugh if you will, in a Japanese accent, which brought my host brother out and he started to laugh also. After his laughter at my expense, he came down and took me to where the bath was. This was a typical Japanese bath, but was heated by fire. It looked like a horse troth, but it was big. I undressed, hung my clothes in the changing area and got in and soaped up. Not finding a drain, I got out and dried off. When I went to get my clothes in the changing room only to see, a Japanese robe waiting for me. I just assumed it was for me to use. Where my clothes went, I would not find out till the next morning. I went into the kitchen to have some café and sat down. My host father went into the hall and was about to take a bath.

Suddenly, I heard what sounded like Japanese swears. Pai Terabe, aka, Papa Terabe, came in and took my hand and led me into the bath area. He proceeded to tell me in sign language or gestures that I was to take a shower first and then soak in the bath. I had just ruined the family bath or soaking tub.

Embarrassed, I decided it was time to go to bed. To get to my room, I had to leave the main house and walk down a long porch where there were several doors to bedrooms that had been the children's rooms for many years. They had all grown up, so they were now empty and used for guests and storage. Entering my room, I did not see my luggage or clothes. I just figured it was another custom and just went to bed. When I woke up, the window was open, and the door was open. My clothes were all laid out, shoes shined, and luggage put aside. I was also lying on the bed with covers gone and I was naked, which is how I went to bed, not having any clothes the night before.

I closed the window and door and got dressed. I went down to have breakfast, and my host mom would not look at me. She just pointed to the coffee. It was very uncomfortable, but I just sat at the table and drank my coffee. My host brother came in and just giggled under his breath. Finally, I asked him what was going on. He told me that it is their custom to wash all the clothes of the guest as illness, germs, and bugs can be carried from house to house. After she washed my clothes, she came to put them in the room in the morning. The door was locked, so she opened the window and reached over to unlock it. She came in and put my clothes away and went to wake me. I did not wake up, so she removed my covers and saw I was naked. She then ran out.

This was my first day and my first experiences in "culture shock." I would experience many more episodes of culture shock, but this one hit home. I began to understand that I was in another culture in someone else's home and that I would need to understand the diversity of culture if I was to survive with some dignity.

After I came back from Brazil, I was a different person. My growth accelerated through my experiences faster than many of my friends. They seemed to have stayed the same as when I left, in most cases. The ego in me wanted to tell everyone about what I had experienced, but the Caregiver in me dictated that I slow down and try to fit into this new, old culture that to me had not changed. It was me who had changed. This was the true culture shock I was not told about. I had to learn about it for myself. Since then I have been working as an Area Rep for several foreign exchange programs where students come to this country. I created and set up a class for them about the culture shock they were not told about, and hoped it would sink in.

My job entailed receiving students from other countries, place them in families in the area, and enroll them in the school in the family's district. It was a stressful year, and I was able to place most of the students from the European countries, but it was more difficult to place the students from Africa and South America for some reason. As the Rep, I had to make sure they had a place to stay, and two of the last to come came from Liberia and Ecuador. Why it was so hard to place them, I do not know and will not speculate. My mom saw the problem and said, "Let them stay here." Not sure if it was a good idea, I was desperate and agreed. The one from Liberia was T. Romeleus Cooper. He was an amazing student who was full of charm, wisdom and fun. My family took to him quickly and vise versa. The year went well, and we did have our ups and downs, but that is what siblings do. He went home to Liberia, and I did not hear much from him for a while.

If you look at African or Liberian history, there was a takeover of the government and a lot of killing, went on. Trampus, (which is what the T in his name stood for), escaped and is now living in Virginia. We have since connected, and one of the things he told me that he missed most about home was that he had to leave all his school stuff from the states and most of his belongings. This got me to think that it would be amazing if I could get his yearbook from school and give it to him. I called the school and was able to acquire one of the last ones they had from that year.

Forty-four years after Trampus left my home, I sent him the one thing that he could connect to who he was when he was a student here-His Yearbook. We have since connected and refer to each other as true brothers. I am so proud to call him family, and I know he is proud to be part of my family.

I have since worked in many situations where I was the only white guy around. Learning how to fit in was an awakening. To be on that side of the coin gave me a new appreciation for the issues that many cultures experience. We live in such a diverse country culturally, and in many cases you can just walk out your front door to experience this. I am lucky; I survived many visits to the projects in NYC where I had to pick up Homer, who is now my son. If I had the van, I had to sit in it till he came down to meet me. When I took the car with the sign in the window that said 'Clergy' I got, "Good morning, Father. Nice day, Father. We will watch your car, Father. Bless you, Father." I think I got a real good look at what the fear of God looks like, or how well-respected God is. When I came back down from Homer's apartment on the top floor, the guys around the car would tell me that they watched my car. I feel a bit guilty, but instead of giving them a tip I gave them my blessing. I hope my counterfeit blessing worked for them.

These moments in my life have prepared me for the caregiving field in many ways, since working with someone who is ill is like meeting someone who is in a different culture. To this day I have learned to respect the differences and diversity of each person I meet and work with. But the main thing I have found is that clear communication, respect, and treating everyone with the dignity I would wish for, is the key to so much in our society and to the success as a Caregiver. You, as the Caregiver, are entering a different world and culture. Treat it that way, and your vision will be filled with a full-color spectrum and appreciation of the cultural diversity we all live in.

THE BED RUN AND MY AMIGO

Mark had been getting progressively sicker. The trips to the doctor's office were getting more frequent. I knew we had to do something about his sleeping arrangements as he was never very comfortable. He would always prefer to lay on the floor with a blanket over him and a pillow under his head and feet. My father had just died, and there was a hospital bed in his house. My first thought was to just go down and get it, but having no truck or van I needed some help. I had a friend, Sal Palazzo, who I had known since the early 70s. We had one of those friendships where we were inseparable.

While I was in Brazil, I learned a little bit about friendship and the difference between friendships here and friendships down there in Brazil. Here we can have many friends and someone I've known for a short time, could be considered a friend. In Brazil, the word for friend is "amigo". If I were to say that you were my amigo, it would mean that we've known each other for a very long time and not much, barring death, could break our friendship. It was an establishment in Brazil that was well protected during my stay there in the 70s. If I just met someone or worked with someone for a little while I could call them "conhecido" or acquaintance. Until we've spent a lot of time working on the friendship, which takes a lot of doing, we can't be considered friends.

I told Sal about this, and he liked the idea, so we made a commitment that we would work on it. This meant that I would have to respect his opinions, even if they were opposite from mine. If I was angry with him or if he was angry with me, we would let each other know, and no matter how far away we were from each other we would try our best to keep in touch. Of course, with Facebook, this is not a challenge anymore.

Sal now lives in Arizona, and we are still considered best friends. Our political views are pretty much the opposite in many cases, but the basic values are the same. We respect each other's opinions and understand each other to the T.

We have been friends now for over 47 years. Every time we get in touch with each other, it's like we never left. That is why in the 1990s I asked him to help me with "the bed run", as I call it. Mark desperately needed a comfortable, workable bed, as his legs were filling up with fluid. He had to raise them many times, and it was a lot of work for him and me. I called Sal and told him about my situation, and he said, "No problem." So, I took a train up to Rhode Island from Connecticut and met him. We went to my father's house, which was hard for me because I had just lost my father. A lot of things were still in place. We walked around the property, and I talked to Sal about a lot of the memories I had. Being a photographer, I also started taking some pictures. It was good to be with Sal again. I knew I could count on him.

Suddenly he said, "We need to get going". I realized it was getting late and he had to drive me to Connecticut and then drive back. So, we got things together, went into the house and pulled out the bed. We loaded it up into the van and off we went.

Sal and I could talk about anything. We had no secrets. We had no fears of each other, and I could trust him fully. Before we hit the road again I thought we should stop to get a bite to eat so we could chat a bit. Conversations were lively, catching up on things and remembering old times. After a good strong cup of coffee, we were on our way. As we drove, we began to have those silent moments we all experience when talking for a long time. I encountered a couple of those, which started my mind going in all kinds of directions. Sal knew I was kind of stressed, so he asked me what was up. I told him about what I was going through with Mark, and how much it has drained me emotionally. He perfectly understood, and we did a lot of talking about how we both had experienced similar things. Suddenly, I mentioned a few things about how much I missed Mark, the old Mark. I didn't know what it was going to be like after he was gone. I started to break down and cry. Sal knew exactly what I was going through. We stopped on the side of the road and took a breather.

I embraced Sal as he gave me his shoulder to cry on. I knew I could count on him for anything. His words, as few as they were, were comforting enough to make me feel better. We got back into the van and moved on, as we wanted to get there as soon as possible.

We got to the apartment house, and I ran up the stairs and into the living room where Mark was laying on the couch with his feet up on the end of it. Sal came in and said hi, and we sat and talked for a few minutes. I told Mark that we had gotten a hospital bed for him. Even though he knew it was coming his facial expressions were more like "Oh no, now I'm up to the point where I have to have a hospital bed." I tried to reassure him that it would be better and we should at least try it and if it doesn't work, I can take it back. He said, "Okay."

Sal and I ran down the stairs to the van and brought up the bed. Mark had seen us bringing it in. I had no idea what was going on in his head. We got it set up, plugged it in and made sure it was working alright. After finishing I suggested going into the living room for a bit. Suddenly, Sal stood up and said "I have got to get going because I have to be back for supper and it's going to be a couple of hours ride". He and Mark said their goodbyes, and I walked with Sal down to the van. I looked at him and said thank you, yet I couldn't thank him enough for all his support.

He told me that he couldn't imagine what I was going through after seeing Mark in person again. I told him it wasn't easy and if it weren't for him, my head would be a mess. He said "Let's keep in touch." So, we did for some time. When Mark passed away, Sal was going through some family matters that needed to be taken care of, so he never made it to the funeral. I didn't mind because I knew he was there in spirit.

After Mark's death, I connected with Sal several times, which gave me a breather from all the chaos. One thing I can suggest to anybody going through the process of caregiving and grief is to find one person you can entirely trust and rely on. Someone you can call up at any time of the night, and there would be no problem and no hard feelings. Someone who you can call up and say "I need to get away" and then make plans to do it. Someone who knows you inside and out. Sal was my rock for so long, and even though I don't see him regularly. Facebook has allowed me to make that adjustment. And even though we disagree on many points in politics, religion and many other aspects of life, he has been the closest person for the longest time I've ever known.

I can't say he is the only one that I can rely on situations like these, as I have made some very good friends in the past. I don't want to discredit that part of my life by celebrating Sal, but in that moment he was there, and I'm sure many of my friends would have also been there if they could have. Yet I am blessed and lucky to have him in my life. Our friendship has taught me so much, and I am grateful for him.

HAPPYNESS, HOPE AND VIVA

I wrote this in 2000, and many experiences had not happened in my life. There were many people to meet. Homer became my son, Burt retired in 2006 and immediately got very sick with diabetes, and I met Nate. Please consider that. I first want to apologize if I am about to offend some of you in the context of using a few words (the R-word to be specific) that were commonly used in the day and because it was part of the name of a group who helped many individuals with disabilities.

Since that time the use of that word has been deemed politically incorrect and rightly so but to get a real sense of the time and place of the events, I have chosen to leave them as they were. Since that time the use of the words Special, Exceptional, Mentally Handicapped and Challenged have been their replacements, only to be criticized by some as just another label. The word Happiness is spelled Happyness for one reason and one reason only. I could not spell for the life of me when I created the camp and it became the brand name. It worked, as it did draw attention and people did ask questions.

A Place Called Happyness

As a young boy, I was considered very shy. There weren't very many kids who were my age in the neighborhood I grew up in. It was usually the same three or four kids I would hang out with. I could also not venture out too far from my yard, which was a one and one-half acre piece of land. It had a few outbuildings including the two garages, a shed that housed chickens and my pigeons, and a large area behind the garages that had enough rabbit coops to house up to 200 bunnies by Easter. They served as income and as a meat source for the year. We weren't wealthy by any means, but were a very close-knit family living above our grandfather on the second and third floors. Most of the clothes I wore as a kid were my cousins' hand me downs or created by my mom who taught me a lot about sewing and keeping clothes in good shape.

When I was about 10 or so, I remember a young boy who was different from all the others in the neighborhood. Some of the neighbor kids called him China Boy due to his facial features, and I would later learn he had Down Syndrome. I did not know what that was, but I did know he was different. A few of the neighbor kids would taunt him and make fun of him. In his innocence, he thought it was a game and laughed when they were laughing at him. This troubled me enough that I wanted to keep him safe, so I became his friend and protector of sorts. This act of friendship would become physically painful for me, as they targeted me as the "Retard's Friend" and would push me and taunt me. I was just happy he was not the one getting hurt. In the back of my mind, I wanted to do something to make a difference and create a place where he would be safe. He eventually moved, and the taunting stopped for both of us. He inspired me so much that it would later cause me to experience caregiving in its purest form, but I would not realize that for another 50 years.

As I got older, my parents felt the need to help me meet more kids my age. Not knowing what to do when I met new kids, I stayed in the background of a lot of events at our church and my school. I began attending camps, 4-H meetings, scouts and other youth groups in the church with a lot of encouragement from Mom and Dad. They, along with my downstairs live-in grandfather, were my greatest support and encouragement to excel in all I did. My grandfather especially made me feel good when I wanted to try something new. He always said that if I wanted to do something, I should look at it from all angles, see what I like and dislike and what the advantages and disadvantages were, and then try it. He also said that if I wanted to do something and didn't try it, I would regret not doing it, but if I tried it and succeeded or failed, I would always know the results and could deal with that accordingly and would have learned some lessons from it along the way. If I did not try, I would never know.

That advice has carried me through to this day. It has allowed me to have experiences I would otherwise not have had in areas I would normally not be involved in, and has given me a wealth of knowledge I would have lost out on had I not at least tried. Still shy and going to all these groups, at least one group per night, Scouts Monday, youth choir rehearsal Tuesday, school night activities Wednesday, 4-H Club Thursday, dances or dance committee Friday, farm chores and family outings Saturday, Church and Youth group Sunday and once a month my grandparents from Massachusetts came down to visit. I did not have much idle time for myself. Now that I look back at it, I wished I had more idle time. I think kids today have much too much time on their hands. I also struggled with my self-esteem, which plagued me through high school and beyond. Yet I was still busy with groups, meetings, and projects.

I had become my father in many ways, as he was a very shy and sickly child, but as an adult he got involved in so many organizations and civic groups. It earned him many awards for his concern for others. Unfortunately, that meant that he was at meetings a lot, but so was I. I had also become my mother, with her caring and giving heart. It is easy to fall prey to those who can take advantage of people with a big heart. We were a close family but a busy one in the community, and even though we had little in the way of monetary wealth, we made up for it in the riches of the heart and giving of ourselves and our talents whenever we could. Both Mom and Dad would bring us to events as a family and showed us firsthand what participation in the community meant.

For some reason, and I believe it was that I was finding my ego, I enjoyed being a part of the community service activities and participating in events, parades, and projects where there were things to do and learn. I became so obsessed with this that it affected my grades tremendously.

Education came in second to community involvement. To compensate for my fears and inhibitions, I excelled in many of the areas I enjoyed and did not partake in things I was unsure of, which was contrary to what the school system policies were. One incident comes to mind. I was asked to be in a play with the youth group. My reading skills were not up to the level that most of the kids were at. It was at an elementary level when I was in junior high, but I could read fast, silently. I am still a slow reader, but I take in more than most, and I am a more visual learner than most. I began to read the part in the play. Suddenly the secret was out, I could not read well. Embarrassed, I ran out of the room. The minister came out to meet me and sat with me. He assured me that no one was laughing at me. They were instead concerned. One of my friends in the group asked if there was anything she could do to help me read better.

I now see how and why I got involved in so many care-oriented and service-oriented programs and did well. I kept myself so busy and achieved so much I began to be recognized as somebody for my accomplishments, contributions, and ability to adapt to many situations, rather than for my academic skills. I also began to receive recognition for my work. I received awards and certificates of achievements. Some of them were the Key Award in 4-H (which is the highest you can get), Outstanding Young Men of America Nominee, was one of eight selected from the US to attend the Canadian National 4-H Convention, and in 1969 I got the Youth of the Year Award given by the Association for Retarded Children at that time. This confirmed my belief that I was doing the right thing and that I was accepted for who I was and what I had done.

Up to that point, my life was all ego. It felt good to receive awards and to hear people recognize me in groups as someone who was doing well. Yet it was still a fragile situation, as failure and criticism were hard for me to swallow, and still are. But I still listened and learned from it all. I learned that it was OK to fail if I knew I had put into it the best I could and had learned something from it.

While I was in High School I had a part-time job as a dishwasher in the old JJ Newberry's store in town. I was so proud to get a minimum wage, which was $1.25 an hour. It had long been a local favorite social gathering place with its long lunch counter. One of the sales ladies, Mrs. Brouseau in the jewelry department, Mrs. Brouseau, was someone I enjoyed talking to and was fun to work with. She always had a pleasant smile, and it was sincere. One evening as I was cleaning the dish area and she had a coffee, she began telling me about a group her daughters Lucile and Diane were getting involved in. It had something to do with mentally challenged individuals. They were a good group of teens, and she felt I would get along well with them.

I had only met one mentally challenged individual when I was eight years old, and as a teenager had used the word "retarded" frequently to describe some of my peers who I was not too fond of. I was under the impression that most mentally challenged individuals were in facilities like Ladd School and Howard, two institutions dealing with mental illness at this time. They no longer exist in that capacity, as most were dismantled and many of the residents were introduced into the community with group homes. I didn't know many individuals were living with their families at home and that there were now community programs for them. I was not sure I wanted to get involved, but she encouraged me to attend. The first meeting the group had was in the old St John's School, a Catholic school in the town where many of my classmates had attended. The school is no longer there. The night of the first meeting came. I came down with the flu and couldn't participate, which kept me from being a charter member. The next meeting was a couple of weeks later, and I made sure I attended that one. There were few familiar faces, but it was a friendly group.

The meeting lasted about an hour, and their group was attending to issues concerning what they would do as a unit to help the children. The name of the group was "Senior Teens Against Retardation" later changed to "Senior Teens Aid Retarded" and nicknamed STAR. It is now called "Senior Teens Assist Recreation" and is still in existence. It does some good work in the community. Unfortunately, it has to be run by an agency now for liability reasons.

The first event I attended was a dance. The theme was the Peanuts Party. Being a pretty good artist, I designed all the Peanuts Characters and cut them out to put around the hall. I created my niche in the group, as I would do a lot of the creative projects and recruited some of my art class friends from school. I still had not met the children yet, and wasn't quite sure what to expect.

I recently attended the 50-year reunion of the group and camp. I missed the 45th reunion because I lost my finger to a table saw, so I was not going to miss this one. Attending this one was an inspiration and emotional awakening I hope to harness. Reminiscing with some of the original members, I began to realize that for the past 50 years we as a group had selfishly protected this amazing experience and it was now time to share it. In the short speech I made as founder and first director of the camp we ran, I addressed this idea with the group and found an overwhelming majority willing to share this journey before there are too few left to share it.

For several days before the Peanuts Party, we worked together on drawing and painting, trying to create a Peanuts environment in the former auto mechanics building and storefront for a Chevy dealer, which had been transformed by the town into a youth center and later closed because of teens abusing it and mismanagement. Its closing weren't so many drugs or so much liquor, although beer was on the scene, it was more about the loud music and teenagers dressing wildly. Times were changing in the 60s, even on the local level. Miniskirts and beads and a few tie-dye tee shirts were the shocks of the day, plus the threat of the draft, Vietnam and drugs on the national scene made the struggle of growing up more ominous.

We finally got it all together and waiting to meet the kids. Several teens were the lookouts, ready to greet them when they came in. Most of them were brought by the parents, but some came by bus. Then, it happened. One of the lookouts yelled, "They're here!" and the group got ready. Suddenly, in came a group of swaying, smiling, eager adults of many shapes and sizes with many unfamiliar sounds, but all happy. There was a feeling of joy I could not understand. There were about 25 of had been contacted by the group. They came from many families in the area. Not a bad start-up number.

I wasn't sure what to do or say and I was as nervous as a first-grader going to class for the first time. Just then, a little guy with a funny sense of humor came over to me like an ambassador and shook my hand, introducing himself. "Hi, I'm Roger. Who are you?" And I said, "I am Bob" to which he responded, "Oh" and turned to the next person. Roger and I would turn out to be the best of buddies for years to come. He was like the star of the show, the center of attention, and reminded me of Bob Hope. His smile and genuineness overwhelmed me and drew me to him. I didn't know it, but he was the same age as me, and even though he was strong and rugged he was still a child at heart. It bothered me that they were referred to like children, as they were mostly adults and deserved some dignity. I did not say anything about my feelings about this for some time, until I had more experience. I felt they were not children, and should be referred to as adult people unless their age dictated otherwise.

That day, Roger and I became great friends. This encounter rekindled the memory of that boy in my neighborhood who I befriended. I found out recently Roger is still living in a group home and is about to turn 70, as am I. He is a testament to how far we have come since the institutions of the 50s and 60s where people like Roger could have been warehoused. He and I hit it off, and I would be his STAR buddy whenever we went to the zoo, bowling, or the movies. I was always proud to be with him in public, and I was ready to defend him in any situation. I also was able to correct him when he was not appropriate, and he did also correct me on several occasions.

This was the beginning of my realization of what all those groups, clubs and organizations I had attended when I was young and all the things my parents taught me were all about. They were about caring; caring for others in situations different from mine. Caring for the community and how it is run. Caring for people who have fallen into unjust situations because of who they are, where they come from, what they believe and what they look like. I started to understand a little more about the world, and greed and personal gain at the expense of others were coming into focus in my life with civil rights and all the political agendas rising to the surface. I began to look at who my friends were and how some of their jokes were at the expense of others. I began to learn how to select my friends based on their beliefs, actions and how they treat others, and not on how they looked or if they were popular. I began to open my eyes more. The main thing was that I began.

As a teen in 1968, I was aware of and sympathetic to a group that was widely misjudged, in my opinion. This was the hippie movement. It was a time that had begun shortly after the Kennedy assassination when people were, into looking at the world differently. The Funeral of Kennedy was one of the first live TV in the US and it was now showing the injustice of how the Black population was being treated. I was not a hippie and yes, I did rebel in some ways, but I didn't cause riots or use drugs or guns. I was being herded into the corral because I was a teenager who thought differently and from all the reports on TV, most teens were hippies on drugs and rebels. At this point, I started to understand what the Black population was talking about, being judged by the color of their skin and who they were as human beings. I listened to programs on TV about how the Jews in WWII in Germany. And even though they tried to express the real magnitude of what happened with little visual evidence, people still doubted them, and that bothered me. Many people did not believe the Holocaust happened and some still don't today. My shyness was still a barrier for me, as my self-esteem hadn't been fully developed. That was about to change as I saw the mentally challenged people were also oppressed and put in a classification that did not allow them to develop to their full potential. After a lot of thought and discussion with others, I was about to challenge the community with a new idea.

I had a friend who was also a member of STAR. His name was Bob, and he was always easy to talk to. I used to go over his parents' house when the meetings were over, or on Sunday when STAR event had ended and discuss world events and just about everything else. I had an idea that I thought would be a good project, and a challenge for the group. Bob and I had both experienced camps of some sort, and he became my wall to bounce ideas off of. I thought it would be neat to have a camp for kids with disabilities and having had the experience as a camp counselor for several years, I felt it would be easy to plan and organize.

I had already visualized the camp, how it would run, and how great it could be. Now it was time to convince others it could be done. Bob and I sat at his kitchen table over coffee and discussed as many aspects of it as we could. He played the devil' s advocate many times. I needed that, or I would not have been able to be realistic. Every so often his mother and father would chime in with a parent's point of view. They were usually positive and supportive, but always let us know that not everyone would be as accepting as they were and that it was going to be a long hard road to get to the point where the camp was a reality. We would need a lot of support from the community, parents, and our peers.

The STAR group had fallen into a rut trying to find things to do, as it was always the same each weekend and there were few challenges. Even though we had over 50 members by now, there never seemed to be enough for everyone to do, and we even split the group into two to make it easier. The group was divided by age. There were the young children from ages 6 to 12 and then the older group from 13 up, which made it easier at events as we could design the activities to accommodate the age factor. We also had joint activities, but there was still something lacking. The original mission was not as visible as it used to be and the lack of challenges let the wind out of our sails, so to speak.

After I left Bob's house one night, I stayed up all night planning and writing everything I would need to make this all happen. I created a Road Map. I drew a road map on a paper on the wall with destinations and goals. It was a good visual way to see where I was at a glance. I still use this tool, even if only in my head or on the computer. I look back at that time and sometimes I wish I still had that same drive. There was so much to consider and to plan for, since I wanted only teenagers to be in charge and have several adults there to oversee the program and of course a nurse. I knew that would lead to more challenges as we needed a registered nurse to comply with the law, as well as for our safety. How I was going to convince the adults, let alone my peers and the community at large that this would work was beyond me, but I knew I had to try. I kept thinking about my Grandfather's advice about choice. The experience I would get from Camp Happyness could last me a lifetime. I didn't realize what that was all about then but now, 50 years later, it is crystal clear.

I had to become a salesman, director, fundraiser and organizer all in the same breath. At the same time, I was going to college and holding a full-time job. Could I do it? My mind wasn't sure, but my heart and soul absolutely were. After many hours of writing and dreaming, I had a plan. I would bring it up to the group and get their response. I didn't know if it would go over, but I had to try. At the first meeting we were to discuss the camp, I had asked for some time at the end of the meeting to talk about my idea and to plant a seed, so to speak, within the group. They agreed, and after one of the longest meetings I had ever attended with this group, I had the floor. By that time the group was not ready to listen to many more things, so I made it brief. I could see they wanted to get out of there as soon as possible.

The meeting was held in the West Warwick Police Station on the second floor, just past the holding cell. That was always a reminder that we had to behave well. Now that I look back, it was a good gesture on the part of the police station to let us use the facility. At least we had their support. We had moved the location of the meeting around so many times, from schools, to fire departments, to social clubs and now to the police station. We couldn't pay rent so we had to use whatever we could get. The meeting ended, and the seed was planted. I knew how hard this project was going to be. I didn't think anyone had listened until the next meeting where there was an onslaught of questions about the camp. Apparently what I said at that first camp meeting had left its mark. The air was heavy with anticipation, curiosity, and excitement I hadn't seen in this group in a while. Now all I had to do is tap into the excitement and enthusiasm and just do it.

I scheduled meetings every week for a few months and set a foundation to build from. I also gave reports to the group in the main STAR meetings. This reinforced the idea and made it evident that we meant business to those who were skeptical. One of the main projects was to find a camp that would have us. This was a challenge, as it was the first time we had to approach the community at large, who had their opinions about teenagers and the mentally handicapped. It was like two strikes against us right at the start. After contacting several camps, I found that by describing the clientele who would be attending, I got nowhere with them. However, by just discussing the use of the facility, it gave us a chance to get through the door. At that point, we were able to see the camp and break down the components and discuss the details, giving us at least a chance to show them who we were. In the end, I approached a total of thirteen camps and finally was able to convince W. Alton Jones Camp, which was headed by the late Mr. Wheatley and was an extension of the University of Rhode Island, that 30 teens could pull it off. I had been involved with 4-H clubs when I was younger and knew some of the people there. If anyone says "it's not who you know but what you know", think again. It's both.

Raising the money became our second priority, because if we couldn't find the money it would not happen. We now knew how much we would need, $2300 to run the camp. Where were 30 teenagers going to get that much money? Car washes and cake sales were only a drop in the bucket, and we had only a few months to go. Our appeal went out to the adult community, who knew us by now. We had made a name for ourselves as responsible teenagers, and that was going to be a plus for us. In the end, we were able to touch the caring side of the adult groups, and they began giving. The Elks Club, the Lions club, Rotary Club, many of the churches, and several individuals all made it happen. That is why I say we are all Caregivers.

At that time, I was asked what the name of the camp was. In the back of my head I had a lot of names that it could be called, but the one I loved was Camp Happyness. I had cards made up and sent out letters with the misspelling of the name. Some were amused by the misspelling of it but most said nothing. When asked why it was spelled that way, I simply admitted I could not spell for beans.

The time came to launch the camp and get the kids there. We had an orientation for two days, and then it was showtime. Camp Happyness lasted a week. It was an overnight camp run by teenagers funded by the community, and appreciated by all who attended. It was an incredible feeling for me to see a dream come true so early in my life. My ego had just received a booster shot, and my level of self-esteem went up. Most of all, I was proud to be with a group of so many caring individuals who were not getting paid for their time and were truly doing it out of love.

The camp is still going on 50 years later in a different form, and has involved many, many teens and community members all over the state. The following year, I had an opportunity to go to Brazil through a program with the 4-H called International 4-H Youth Exchange. This meant that after three years of creating, struggling, building and executing the camp as founder and director, I had to cut the cord. The hardest thing I have ever had to do was to let go and let the new order run my baby. Like a true father, I protected it to the fullest. I later watched all that went on while I was in Brazil, knowing I left it in good hands. It was truly a success. It ran without me. My time in Brazil was filled with new experiences and founding new programs, but a piece of my heart was left at the camp. I got to see it succeed at a distance. One of the letters I received while in Brazil was from the camp, and it was written on a paper towel and signed by everyone at the camp to say thank you for caring enough to create the idea of Camp Happyness. The saying, "if you love something, let it go" rings true here but I must add, if it continues without you, you did it right.

After I came back from Brazil, I stayed involved with the camp for a few years. One of the rules of the camp was that adults could only work as advisors and not supervisors. In other words, we could only advise the directors and watch. This meant that I could only attend and give my feedback, which was fine with me. To witness the success of a dream completed is an opportunity few people get. I finally saw that I had to back away and allow it to continue without me. If it continued without me, it was a confirmation that it was truly a success and would continue with the right people.

Since those early years, the government regulations and rules will not allow teens to have so much control anymore, and with all the red tape and insurance issues it is a good thing as I did not have those worries and could just concentrate on creating and running the camp. Now with the number of liability cases and "legal stuff," it is an issue that must be attended to by adults.

Hope

Many years after creating Camp Happyness, I was approached by a nurse at Rhode Island Hospital in Providence, while my father lay in a comam, about a camp for kids in the area who had cancer, Camp Hope. I knew her from high school, so we had some connection before this. She was attending to my father as he lay there in a coma had spoken to me about this camp, which was held each year for children they knew who had cancer and their siblings. She knew about my experience with Camp Happyness, so she was eager to talk to me. I wasn't sure about attending it, as my father was still in a coma and Mark was still sick, and my job as a Caregiver was in full swing. We discussed the similarities between the two camps and how they give hope and enjoyment to many kids who need a place where they could feel accepted and normal. I saw this as a vital component in anyone's recovery and growth, whether it be from an illness, addiction, or the death of a loved one.

My father's death in the spring of 1992 and Mark's death in late July gave me a chance to look at the possibility of attending her camp. It was funded by the Rhode Island Cancer Society and was well run from what I heard. I wasn't sure if it was the right thing to do so soon after the deaths of two loved ones, but I decided to give it a shot and called her. I spoke to her about the camp a bit more and told her to hold a place for me. I wanted to help. I didn't know what a healing experience it would turn out to be or how hard it would be on my emotions, but it was something I felt I had to do. She knew I was a photographer and that I did slideshows to music.

The day came when I was to head for the camp. The drive up to Rhode Island from Stamford was filled with mixed emotions and many thoughts zipping through my head. I thought a lot about Mark and all the time I had spent as his Caregiver and Dad's experience in the intensive care unit, as they were fresh on my mind. I kept thinking of some of the funny things that had happened while in the intensive care unit, like the time my cousin Joan came in, who worked for an ICU. She lifted his eyelids and noticed that his eyes were moving slowly back and forth. Her comment was, "I had a clock like that once." It broke up the moment and made us all feel at ease. Questions like, "Will I be able to get through the week without breaking down?" and "Will they accept me even though I am an outsider?" were coming up, along with a host of others.

When I arrived at the campground, I found that I had already acquired a new nickname. "What about Bob?" would be heard at events throughout the week, such as when I would get to a meal late, or if I was introduced at an event. My first reaction was the same fear I had when I attended my first camp as a child.

As the day went on and the counselor orientation continued, I felt more and more accepted. It looked as if it was going to be fun and a great way to get away from all that was happening at home. I had the chance to talk to a lot of the counselors and discuss their connections to Cancer. Many stories were familiar to me, but so individual and personal.

Mark had Kaposi's Sarcoma (which is a form of Cancer) and had gone through radiation treatments. So, some of the experiences were somewhat familiar, and I began to feel like I was part of the family. I wasn't prepared for the joy and the liveliness of the counselors that were at the orientation. I had just experienced a personal tragedy and saw all the pain Mark had to endure, along with the pain my family had to go through with my father's death and all the uncertainty of him being in a coma. And now I was experiencing joy? Go figure. My job was to be the photographer for the camp, and I offered my services with a slide show at the end of the week, complete with music and tears of joy.

Sunday came, and the campers began to arrive. Piles of luggage were being transported to the cabins, and the body language of old friends being reacquainted was evident. My camera was ready, but I wasn't. It seemed like I needed permission to record what I was seeing. As I got to meet the kids and some of their parents, it was evident that it was okay for me to take pictures. When they saw the camera, they all lined up in a group and posing for the camera which is all the permission I would need. The camp had control of the release forms and the pictures, so I didn't have to worry. It would not limit my creativity with my lens.

The activities and friendships I witnessed there were powerful. I began to feel like part of the family. One such moment was when we all attended a campfire, and we had been singing songs. I was tired and began to zone out with the fire and the background music of the kids singing. It was like when I used to watch television when I was a kid, in a room full of people. Suddenly I would come back to reality, and everyone had left the room. This time I must have been hypnotized by the dancing fire and the music. Suddenly I felt a tap on my shoulder. It was one of the kids. "Hi, I am Eric," he said. He asked me if I was okay. I was shocked to see most of the kids had gone to the main lodge. He asked me if he could sit there and ask some questions about my camera. Having this camera was like having a dog. People loved to talk about it, and it became a conversation piece.

I had been thinking about Mark that night. Eric asked me how I was doing and told him I was thinking about a friend I had just recently lost. He said, "Yeah, mostly everyone here has lost someone or is fighting cancer." At that point, I wasn't sure if I should talk to him about this. I was assured it was okay as he began to tell me how he lost his brother to Cancer and what he felt like. It was such a sobering moment. I found someone who understood what I was going through, and someone who had experienced similar things at a much younger age.

He became my guide, friend, and support for the rest of the week. I even let him use my camera a few times, which was my way of saying thank you. I began seeing things a little differently through kids like him and the others. I had just gone through the experience of seeing someone I love go through pain, suffering and death. What I was now seeing was a lighter side of this thing called cancer and grief through the eyes of these young individuals. They were laughing and playing just like other children, but also going through the same pain and suffering that Mark and I felt. With cancer there seems to be a little more hope involved, hence the name Camp Hope, whereas AIDS didn't have much hope at all.

My outlook was a little brighter now because of the smiling faces and their words of comfort, which I still carry with me. Taking life one day at a time was my main lesson. No matter what the problem might be, if I just take life one day at a time, things have a way of becoming workable. They may never work out, but they are workable. Life is beautiful if we just look at it in the present, with a side of humor and a chuckle. Children live life with a very limited past and an undefined future. They live in the present.

After camp was over, I drove to my father's house, which was now somewhat empty, and saw my past as it was now in the present. It was okay. As I drove home to Connecticut, I began to reflect on all the joy and wonderful things we had experienced together. I also thought about the future, which would now be different because of the amazing kids and counselors at the camp. We all need a wake-up call, and this was mine. Remembering the times when Mark and I would live for the moment and take advantage of the times when things weren't too bad made me realize that I had been living in the present all along. After Mark's death and the death of my father, I felt all I had was the past with all its memories and "shoulda, coulda, woulda" moments. When I got home, I took stock of what was now my present and began to enjoy it the best I could.

Sure, there were low points, and I knew they would happen, but they were also what allowed me to deal with them in the present. After six months, living in the present means getting help and support. Doing it by myself was no longer an option. Now, hope is a real thing to me. In my work with AIDS programs, I try to convey to the client the idea that they are still here, and they are living now. Of course, it is always "now" and it is still hard to deal with for those who are HIV positive and those who are affected, (meaning parents, spouses, families, and friends). But if I can give them a little glimmer of happiness with a smile or the realization that the present is important too, I have served them well.

At the end of the camp, I took all the pictures and turned them into slides. We did not have the technology back then to use computers, so it was a real "slide show". I put it to music, and all the kids sat on the beach with a campfire. The music came from the loudspeakers at the main hall, so it echoed through the woods and across the pond. They got to see themselves during the week through my eyes, and a chance to see how they have changed on a suspended white sheet on the beach. What these kids gave me in a week would and has lasted a lifetime. I am better for it, and I hope they feel they got something out of what I had to offer them. I did meet one of the kids in a seminar many years later, and he said that the one thing that stuck in his mind for many years was being able to see himself in that slideshow with music and know his life was good. He thanked me, and I said: "No, thank you for letting me do it."

Viva

In 1995, I was working for a program called the Upper Room which was primarily geared to helping People with HIV. It was under the umbrella of The Sharing Community. It was my job to teach people who were HIV positive to act as Peer Educators in the community. They would be invited to talk about the illness and how to be safe. It was called the Upper Room because of the disciples who used an upper room in a building to meet and discuss the day's events with Jesus. The Upper Room was designed to be a safe place for people with HIV/AIDS to get together, learn about new breakthroughs, and get access to support groups in the community. I had heard about a camp being organized which would be available to families and individuals affected by or infected with the AIDS virus. I remembered how it was for me when I finally found a place where I could discuss the issues I was facing as a grieving Caregiver without fear of judgment, and how important it was for the kids at Camp Hope.

The camp was called Camp VIVA and I asked how I could get involved. After losing Mark and several other friends to AIDS, I needed to do something positive that was connected to the virus and helped the community. I could see how important it could be for someone with the virus or their family to have a place like this camp to go and feel a sense of normalcy. I was committed to doing what I could to help get it going. I was very familiar with starting a camp because of my previous experience as the founder of Camp Happyness. I got so caught up in the beginning, getting it organized and all, that it began to affect my job, even though my job was dealing with the same population on a community level. Being the Peer Educator for the Sharing Community, which Rev. S Burtner Ulrich (or Burt) and Rev. John P Duffell co-founded, my job was to form peer education groups to educate others about HIV/AIDS. With funding in the New York area becoming so uncertain and with so much work to do, I could not take much time out from my job to do pre-camp activities. As much as I wanted to help form the structure of the camp and be involved, I couldn't put the amount of time and effort I wanted to into it, and decided to just be a part of the camp itself.

I offered my services as a photographer to record the events of the camp on film from its inception and give everyone involved the opportunity to see themselves in action. I was known for setting my slideshows to music, so I had in the back of my head the idea that at the end of camp I could produce a slideshow about the week everyone had just experienced. Even though I would become a photographer, I was also a counselor who had responsibility for three boys around the age of 13. This was going to be a challenge, but I was ready. The orientation was pointing more toward sensitivity training and understanding all the uncertainties and issues that can surround people living with this virus, or living with someone with the virus. I got a chance to really explore the knowledge from my experiences with the virus and use what I knew in a real life setting for education, recreation, and just living life. There were many people at camp from all walks of life and all levels of experience with this virus. Some of the counselors freely disclosed they were HIV positive, which was wonderful, since they gave people who hadn't had much contact with those who were HIV positive a chance to ask questions freely and get answers first hand.

It became quite a community. We all were volunteering our time to do this. After the orientation, it was time for the campers to enter. This would not be the traditional camp with a lot of kids. This was a camp where whole families could experience a place that was safe and supportive. They came in busloads from all parts of Westchester. I saw some familiar faces, and this was the first time I would be with them outside of my work in Yonkers. I was introduced to the boys I would be caring for, and at that point I was ready for anything, but I didn't know what I was in for. I was introduced to the first one, Daryl (for confidentiality reasons, I have changed the names of my campers), who was taller than me, bigger than me, and was not going to cooperate if he did not have to. We were all about to stand in a circle and hold hands to sing the camp song. He was standing next to me. As I reached for his hand he said, "I don't hold hands," and proceeded to fold his arms. I thought to myself, "it looks like we are going to have an interesting week together", but I was glad he was able to express his feelings in any case.

I then met my second camper, Eddie, who was a bright, intelligent and articulate 13-year-old who I found out later had written a published book. He turned out to be one of my inspirations while writing this book. I felt we had something in common and hoped we would get along. Then there was my third camper, Ben. He was a wiry kid who was introduced to me by his Mom, who I knew. She had to hold onto him so I could meet him. I reached out to shake hands, and he got away from his Mom and went to kick a soccer ball that just went by. His foot connected with my shin, which slowed me down for the rest of the week. When I met him in the circle, he slapped me five and gave me a smile like nothing had happened. I later found out that the littlest things would set him off, and he would go into a rage. Just a normal kid from New York.

There I was, three entirely different personalities with egos, a wild side, and me with a camera. Ben's Mom and I became good friends, and she taught me about growing up black in the projects. I didn't pretend to understand much of their culture, as she opened my eyes to it.

The first part of the week was tough, as we were all functioning on a power struggle. There were a few words exchanged and a few fists that flew. The organizers at the camp were well prepared for any of these unscheduled events that would pop up every so often. They all acted professionally, and I truly have the utmost respect for all of them. My three campers slept in the same room with me, which meant I had to go to sleep long after they did because I snore. That secret did not last very long, and I began to be on the receiving end of snoring jokes and gestures. It wasn't until I made a joke at myself about the snoring that they began to respect me about my night music.

Sharing the same room with them made it easy to have a captive audience. We would sit together before we turned on the TV (I know, TV at camp? It was an urban camp!) Anyway, it gave us some time to talk about the day and answer any questions they might have about anything. We talked about basketball, what others did to irritate them, swimming, and any issues that came up including girls and all the problems they were experiencing communicating with the opposite sex. I wasn't Dr. Ruth, but I did provide another point of view. They were not afraid to say what they thought, which made me realize I had made a breakthrough. Even though there were serious concerns, they made them jokes, as a defense mechanism I suppose. There were some poignant and heartwarming discussions woven in this quilt of teenage testosterone.

Several days into camp life, the temperature was in the 90s that day and tempers flaring on the basketball court. The kids were just about to finish the game when one of them thought he got ripped off taking a shot. He began yelling at the others. Ben was not in on it but decided that he would try to put in his two cents. He was really angry, and I knew I had to get him away from the others for a while. He resisted, and I lifted him by the belt and guided him through the gate where the court ended. 1 asked the counselors there to watch the others while I took him for a walk.

I took him down toward the pond, and we walked around the pond for about an hour without a word. I was afraid he might think he was in trouble, so I asked a few questions but still got no response. I knew he was angry about a lot of things and could not talk about them, so I just backed off. As we walked, I would stop to skip some rocks across the water. He tried skipping some but was not doing well, so I showed him how to hold it and throw it. He tried, and I guess that broke the ice as the word "sick" eked out. (Sick, I found out later, meant cool). We walked a while longer and chased the geese (of which there were no shortages). When we got to the beach, I noticed he was wearing my sneakers and had my Vermont Cow cap on. Since I had my camera and was behind him, I took a picture. The sun was setting, and it was a perfect shot.

We sat on the beach, and suddenly he asked me, "Do you like me?" This question caught me off guard a bit, so I said, "Well, what is there about you that I could learn so I can have more information to go on?" He said, "I don't know, I get angry a lot and people don't like me." I said, "I like you and think you are a great kid, so maybe you could think about all the good things there are about you, and you tell me what they are. What is there about you I would like?" He sat for a while and then said, "OK, but I need to think about it," and I said, "Sure." Before we got up to leave, he said thanks for letting him use my hat all week.

To me, that was quite a breakthrough for Ben. I said, "you can keep the hat if you can think of all the good things that made you who you are", and we shook on it. I also asked if he could cool it on the language and anger. His response was at first more visual with his face, and then he said, "Now you are pushing it." So I said, "How about if you feel like you are getting mad, we can talk?" He said, "OK."

The walk back to the group was nice, and we talked about what we were going to do for the rest of the week. From that point on I was his mentor. He had found a friend at Camp Viva.

The next day we were at lunch, and he asked me if he could talk to me. I said, "Sure." He wanted me to sit at a certain table. I told him I had planned on sitting at another table with someone, but he insisted I sit with him. He began asking if I wanted coffee. I told him I would have some after I ate but he again insisted I have coffee now. The cup at each place setting was upside down on the saucer. As he went to get a pot of coffee, I turned the cup over. A folded piece of paper fell out. It was a list of all the good things about being Ben. Some were corny, but most were sincere. His biggest asset was his smile, and I confirmed them all and told him that this was the Ben I liked. I later gave it to his mom and, yeah, you guessed it - tears.

When we got back to the group, I could sense some jealousy going on, so I had to make a point of paying equal attention to the other two. Eddie was a pretty matter-of-fact guy who was quite independent. I had thought I would have connected with him more than the others, as he had a very creative mind. He did command more attention from his peers than adults, so I pulled back a bit. However, Daryl was not a happy kid. He was slowly getting more and more frustrated and angry with little things, and it began to affect the group as a whole. I noticed he had an interest in cameras, since he was always looking through my camera bag. He loved looking through the telescopic lenses. I decided I would give him some film and let him use one of my older cameras. We sat and talked about the cameras and how they worked, and for the first time I had his full undivided attention, and he was listening. As I have said before, if you want to work with kids, find out what their passion could be, and you are good to go. At first I let him use the small lenses and then, when he felt comfortable, I let him use the "big guns" as he called them, the telephoto lens. With this lens, he could zoom in on things far away and explore things that were out of reach. Because he was thirteen, I also had to monitor where he was looking, as I caught him looking at the girl's dorm. It was pretty obvious he was watching something he liked. He had a smile a mile-long on his face.

Over the next three days he gained a new vision of the world and his surroundings. He became curious, asked questions, and began to laugh and make jokes that were not hurting others. He reminded me of myself when I had my first camera and began to see the world in different ways. I had forgotten that exploratory part of my life. He also helped me see how far I have come, from the anger I experienced when I lost Mark and all the other people who had died from complications from HIV, cancer, and life. Even with all the pain around us, he showed me how beautiful life still was. He had also lost someone with HIV, so we had a common thread there.

The last night at the camp was a special night for all. There was a talent show and a celebration. Then the lights went out, and I began to show my slideshow. Everyone got to see so many pictures of themselves from just a few days before, and got to see how much they had changed. The music was the kicker, and there was not a dry eye in the house. My Three Musketeers came up to me and hugged me for the first time all week. Wow! What a breakthrough, and what an experience that was. The parents and many of the counselors were moved and said that it was not until the slideshow that they realized how profound this week was.

The last night we were at camp the four of us went up to their room, which they called the loft, or sometimes the pigpen. They were obviously not ready for the good housekeeping seal of approval. We talked about all the things that had happened at camp and all the feelings they had and how they changed. They all had their differences and power struggles, but they were all friends this week. They made a pact that night to stay friends and then proceeded to watch Basketball on TV. They had come such a long way. So, I told them they could stay up as long as they were quiet. That lasted about 30 minutes. The guys in the room next door used a little compassionate kidding around, which would have ended in a battle a week ago. Within an hour all was quiet, and I went in and turned off the TV.

The next day was the hardest day for all of us. We had to leave. Even Daryl had a tear or two. Ben came in as I was packing and gave me a clay pencil holder he had made in the craft class. I gave him the cow hat he had worn all week. Eddie and I talked about the book he wrote and asked me about this book which was in the early stages at that time.

This camp changed the lives of three young men in less than 7 days. I am sure it changed everyone who attended the camp, but I got to witness the transformation of these three individuals. During the week they got to meet James Earl Jones, have fun, and got to witness their transformation through the slideshow of their activities, tears, and successes.

As I look back at my week at Camp Viva, I have fond memories. Since then, one counselor was ordained a minister, many of the kids have gotten married and had their own kids, many have died (including Ben's Mom and Eddie). Some lives have gotten better and some worse, and Ben found out I lived only a few streets away. I can say, he turned out fine.

The camp had a song. The tune escapes me, but the words are engraved in my mind as it was such a great week:

Camp VIVA
We love you
We'll always remember,
This summer and all of the fun

Camp VIVA
We know that
There's more than a week here.
Our friendships have only begun

We're there for each other
In good times and bad
For anything under the sun

Camp VIVA
We thank you
For all of the memories
Together we'll always be one.

When I first heard these words, I didn't know what they would mean until I started writing about the camp. Of course, we would remember all the memories and all the fun. What I didn't realize was that it was truly more than a week at camp. It was the beginning of a lot of friendships that would last a long time. I also didn't realize how much we would truly be there for each other in bad and good times. We became an extended family.

The friendships that came out of that camp were deep. I especially my relationship with Ben, his sister and his mother. Also, many of the counselors have been a positive influence in my life. I grew from their love and concern for each other. With all the events that followed and our united efforts to raise money for more programs and camps, it gave me a new focus. After Mark's death, I knew things were going to be different. Having survived the pain, prejudice, and ignorance about AIDS in the community, I thought everything would be fine. I find myself now sometimes angrier than I was when I was Mark's Caregiver, possibly because of my silence as well as the silence of others.

Now working with a provider group, I see, experience and feel more each day I meet someone new who is going through the same things Mark and I went through in 1992. If I had one wish, I think it would be to not have any reason to write this book. That would mean that AIDS would not be an issue and there would be more tolerance in diversity, understanding, and urgency for people with life changing illnesses, and their Caregivers so they can seek help without being afraid. If you must read this book to heal, it has not happened yet.

I wrote this around 2000. There were many people I would meet. Burt retired in 2006 and immediately got very sick with his diabetes, lost both his legs and died in 2012, and I met Nate who I have been a PCA for 20+ years.

After losing contact with Tony Lembeck and Michael Moffatt since 1999, who were two of the original founding members of Camp VIVA, it was good to catch up. They both are still directing it and they said,

"It is amazing to look back at the beginning and see what a gift we have given so many people just by having the camp." Thank you Tony and Michael for your dedication on behalf of all the campers.

"Haven't Got Time For The Pain"

I believe it was Carly Simon who sang the song with this title. It never meant much to me until lately. Sometime after Mark's death, I began looking at how before, during and after his death, I desperately tried to avoid the pain I was going through emotionally.

Before his death, I was on automatic or autopilot, meaning I was just doing what needed to be done at that moment. It is a safety mechanism that is truly hard to describe, much less explain. A lot of this "automaticness" was to avoid pain. Being upset at times went along with the process of caring for Mark, but was sometimes put aside for many reasons. One of the reasons was that if I began dealing with my pain, I wouldn't have time for his pain and the care he needed. That was what I thought. Looking back, I wish I had dealt with it when it was happening. Of course, we seem to see clearer after things are over. Sort of "Hindsight is 20/20."

Unfortunately, I have carried the "It's Not About Me Syndrome" with me to this day and at times find I don't deal with my pain when I am hurting. I am learning. However, there are still many situations where I find no time for the pain. Pain hurts whether it is emotional or physical. Pain is not what we want in our life, It also can affect the decisions we make.

I can understand how the opiate problem, these days, has exploded. Pain is uncomfortable, pain is an inconvenience, pain comes in many shapes and sizes. In this society where instant gratification is an issue and there is a pill for everything, we need to relieve the pain in any way we can. In 2014 I went to the Select Board in Randolph, Vermont and stood up, declaring that I will not sit down and shut up until someone will listen and agree to discuss the issue of Opiate abuse. I had decided that it was time, after 20 years of asking, to create a forum that could start a conversation about this epidemic. With the growing number of overdoses and deaths in the community, it is time we did something. This eventually led to the formation of the Randolph Opiate Response Team. We now have one of the most aggressive, yet sensitive, groups, which have been listening to the community rather than dictating what needs to be done.

There was also a time when I was so used to pain and not dealing with it, I didn't know what to do without it. Not dealing with it does not mean it goes away, or you don't feel it. It became an old friend I hadn't seen in a while because I ignored it. It was like learning how to deal with it all over again. I would sweep things under the rug and hope they disappeared. They sometimes feel like potholes along the road to wellness. I have tried to fill the potholes with this book and other things. I have to say it has helped.

I often wonder if I would do it all over again, even knowing what I know now. Working in the field with PWA (people with AIDS), I have had to deal with death, grief, and recovery a few times. Even though their deaths affected me, they were not so closely connected, so it was easier to deal with and seemingly quicker for me. At times I feel I am getting numb to death and dying. I truly hope not. It has been quite a few years since I lost Mark and started writing this book. I still grieve, but I have learned how to. One of my colleagues called it "grieving appropriately", meaning grieving the way that is best for me.

The social norm expects us to grieve in a certain way, and can have its limitations. In the beginning, it is OK to cry, yell, feel weak, not quite have all your senses intact or just do crazy things. The period for this is short (only a few days to a week usually) depending on how the death occurred. After that we are allowed to be quiet within ourselves, cry alone, or with loved ones and close friends as long as they understand. This can be allowed to go on for up to a year, but mostly on holidays and birthdays. After that, it's everyone for themselves. If you grieve in public, you could hear pity or the usual, "you should be over this by now", but many times not to your face.

Indeed, it is a lonely road. At this point, it seems appropriate to not have time for the pain. Unfortunately, it can still hurt just as much, but in smaller spurts. Little things can and will trigger your emotions, like a song, a poem, a flower, a place, or just a sunset that looked like the one Mark and I sat and watched in Cancun.

For me, during these spurts, it was easy to assume that life is cruel. Fortunately, I have been able to turn the pain into joy. Sure, I cry, but it is like crying at the end of a wonderfully emotional movie. For many years it seemed unreal to me that he was gone. However his mother and stepfather's, grief is a bit different. It is deeper, and it may take them many years to get to the point where I am now. I understand this, so when their grief shows up, I welcome it and allow it to be there.

These school shootings where the victims are so young and fragile, I cannot imagine the grief the survivors will have to endure. We as a society have to do everything we can to allow their grief, no matter how uncomfortable. As we have seen in the news, it can show up as anger, hatred, and frustration that nothing is being done quick enough. We also have to start the conversation to end these tragedies. Unfortunately, with all the factions and belief systems fighting each other, both socially and politically, it is going to take a very long time.

We will all be at some point in our lives in a grieving state at some point in our lives. Sadly, there is no manual for doing it right or well. If there were such a manual, I would hope to have found it by now. We can make suggestions in books, articles, and research literature, but it still boils down to the individual who is in grief, and only they can know what is right for them.

Through all of this, I found out is that my grief is my own and no one else's. I have the opportunity to own it and mold it into what I feel comfortable with. I know that now, yet I am always afraid that I might forget about owning it while in the autopilot state caring for someone, and I will have to start all over again. It really is like a roller coaster ride. You might see it in this book, where I am positive about life one paragraph and in the next paragraph I am in a slump. This was not on purpose, that was real. The key is to turn it into an adventure and a wonderful learning tool. It can also be an awakening, as it has been for me. I have spent most of my life not seeing all there is to see around me. I still don't, but at times I take off the blinders. I can see pain, hate, sadness, illness, and corruption, but now I also see more of the joy and the excitement that lies between the lines. Sure, many times these things are hard to see, but now that I know they are there I can take the opportunity to at least look. I also have realized that grieving is a selfish emotion. We usually do not grieve an individual's death; we grieve our loss of the relationship and experiences we had with this person. We are more upset or angry about the death part.

Many of the people I have met since Mark's illness have shown me this. I have learned that life doesn't move in a straight line; it also swirls and turns and has ups and downs. Yes, just like a roller coaster.

If I should be so bold to give advice, enjoy the ride. Maybe I'll see you at the end in some way.

NATE

In 1998 I was working at a small school in Vermont. How small? The graduating class that year had only 22 students. Yes, 22. I was working as a para educator in the Special Education division. I had been working with several students who were, let's just say, not enthusiastic about school or the educational system in general. In fact, they reminded me of myself when I was in school. I was one of those students who could only go so far, not being able to complete the task. When I took tests, I could get maybe ten questions done, and then my brain could not wrap around the task anymore. I would literally shut down.

Now they would have diagnosed me with ADD, or even ADHD, which was not a diagnosis then. I was one of the lucky ones though. One of my guidance counselors was able to see what was happening to me and as he once said he was much like me when he was in school. He had to learn how to cope with it in and out of school. What he did to help me was groundbreaking then and changed my life forever.

He took me under his wing, and for the first time I excelled in all my classes. He even gave me rules when I studied. I was to study until I could not focus, and then I was to do something unrelated. To this day I do everything like this, including working with the students. If I need to take a break while working with them, I let them know why and we take a quick walk. When we get back, we continue. The only downside is that now I have so many projects going at the same time, it looks like chaos to others. To me, it is ordered.

Since then I began work in another Vermont school with kids who have it ten times worse than I ever had it. As far as distractions from phones, noise, etc. and the family and social life they have is so broken down, they may seem hopeless. These are the ones I prefer. I always refer to the days I had my counselor's support he graciously took me under his wing and taught me how to teach these kids who no one else wants in their classes.

While working in Special Ed, I met a student who was in a wheelchair and was diagnosed with Cerebral Palsy. I was asked if I would like to work with him as his para educator (now known as the educational technician). Marilyn, who had been working with him since he started school, decided to move on and is now a Special Ed teacher in the same school. She also is one of the most amazing and poised individuals I have ever met. I worked with her twin boys William and Michael in the 7th grade. Michael would eventually assist me in caring for Burt by sitting with him every evening while I was working at night. I can't thank him enough.

I was tossed between working with Nate, which I was familiar with as I had done a lot of work with disabled individuals or with Downs, and working with these other kids who had ADD and could use my knowledge and experience. But when I met Nate, it was a match made in heaven. We hit it off immediately. He liked my jokes and enjoyed my company. This was a kid who may have had 12 vocabulary words tops, could not walk without assistance, and had little control of his extremities. This was going to be a challenge.

I truly enjoyed the first few weeks working with him as he always had a smile and loved to interact with the other kids, many of whom he had known for years. This was going to work, and I was going to make sure it did. As time went on though, I found myself getting tired quicker, and with trying to keep up with his hygiene schedule and taking notes about his health, feeding him at lunch, and all the work I had to do with him, was physically demanding.

However, because he was the only one in the school with this much of a disability there was not much training, support, and guidance. When I asked what I should do with him, their response was, "There is a room down the hall with a lot of his stuff like a Dynavox, a computerized communication device (which needed programming) and teaching aids. See what you can do with that and let me know how you do." I knew I was on my own.

Days, weeks, and months went by, and I was grasping at straws trying to make sense of this. Yet Nate and I were having a blast. He was 12 years old and had charm that would take him far. He used his charm when we would take a walk to the office where Janet, the school receptionist, would take time out every time we went to sit and chat. I knew this would be good as she made sure I did not answer for him and she would wait till he did. Social skills were one of the pieces of his curriculum. He would be asked to do errands like taking notes to the other teachers (as there was no intercom) and taking the lunch counts to the cafeteria.

I knew I could count on the other kids I had worked with, who were usually ready and willing to help me with him, and that made him a star. I would ask one of them to please take Nate to the office, giving them a sense of trust and responsibility, something lacking in the lives of many teens today. I have many former students who still connect with me on Facebook and by email, and they come over to help with the house and remind me of the days with Nate and how that changed them.

Dan Newell was a student who used to mimic Nate was in the hall one day and was making fun of him. I went over to him and told him I was not happy seeing what he was doing and that if he kept it up, I would have to write him up. He continued, and yes, I wrote him up. He was upset with me, and it continued. One day, I saw that he was about to mimic Nate and I walked over to him. I asked him if he wanted to make Nate laugh. He gave me a weird look and laughed at me. I said, "I am serious." So, he said "Sure." I told him to go over to him and whisper in his ear the word "bullshit." He just walked away. I then said

"I dare you." Knowing he would like a challenge, I dared him again, and he finally said, "OK."

He walked over to Nate (who was not happy as this guy was the guy who bullied him earlier). The student leaned over to Nate's ear and said the magic words. Well, Nate could hardly contain himself, and laughed at the top of his lungs, his small, frail body jolting with laughter. Dan could not believe it and did it again, and again he laughed. From then on, until his senior year, Nate and Dan were friends. I could then trust him with Nate. He would ask me if he could take Nate for a walk, and I knew he would be safe. He would even nab him when I was not looking to take him to a class and wait for me to come looking for them, which Nate thought was the funniest thing ever.

With Nate, I spent most of the time working on social interactions, such as how to answer people with the limited vocabulary he had. The Dynavox was not a success, as it took too long for him to find the response and he was very impatient and frustrated. I became his link to conversation and would simplify the request or question for him so the response could be "yes", "no" or "I don't know the answer". It worked for him, and he was happy. His vocabulary increased, and he was able to have limited conversations with others.

While I was working with him in school, I was able to meet his family. Mom was a dynamo who got her way with just a look, and she had to. She had four kids of her own and six others who were adopted, and one from her husband's previous marriage. Her house was run with precision and compassion with so much love it could smother you at times. My time with them was wonderful, and she invited me for supper many times.

One day she asked if I would be willing to be a PCA for a boy with spina bifida who was at times a handful, but a joy to work with. I accepted, and this began my work with her family and Nate. Even though I was Zach's PCA, I was also assisting with Nate, helping feed him, change him, and all those chores we Caregivers must accept as part of the job. Before long I was working seven evenings a week with some weekends off so I could go to New York to help my friend Burt. My social life became limited, but it was ok. The joy that Nate exuded was enough to compensate for any loss in my social calendar.

I began working seven days a week with some of the most enjoyable people I've ever met. Nate and his family were so welcoming. I would get him up at 7:30 A.M. and get him ready for school some days, and I loaded him into his van and took him and Zach to school. There I would be his Special Ed para educator, which meant I spent the whole day with him. One of the problems I found with the school system was that because Nathan was the only one in a wheelchair at the time other than Zach, who's accommodations were limited. I don't believe some of the teachers understood my role with him, so it became difficult to communicate in some ways. We finally got a dedicated room for him, however, it only lasted a couple of years and then we were exiled to the hallway for some time. Finally, we were given a closet near the gym that used to be an office that was about 10 by 7, if that, and housed only a few items that he could use in there. When offices became scarce, we were asked to come up with an idea of how we could use some barriers (which to me would have been too distracting for Nathan to do any sort of learning or concentration) and put them in the entrance of the elementary side of the school. Time went by and his mother Nancy got frustrated enough that she decided we would go in only in the morning and we would continue classes after lunch at his house, which worked out well for me. After school was over, I stayed with him until 8 or 9 at night, depending on what was happening that day. Weekends I would work unless I had to go to New York, or had other things to do. I would also fill in when they had to attend events on the weekends.

Zach was also a member of that family through Foster Care. He had spina bifida and was in a wheelchair part of the time and crutches the rest. He was an amazing young man, brilliant, and loved to sports, mostly baseball. Zach and Nate were inseparable most of the time and were best buddies. Nate was about 12 or 13, and Zack was a little younger. For many years I worked with Nate in the school until he graduated and then continued as his PCA after school to the present time, at his ripe old age of 33. I have worked with him for approximately 21 years.

In about 2008 his father passed away tragically, which was very difficult for Nathan and his family. The stress was hard on his mother, so she moved to another town in Vermont where there were more activities and his social encounters more numerous for Nate. Being the ladies' man he was, he began to make friends wherever he went. It was a good diversion for him, since his father's death and not being in the old house where the memories was a new start for him. He still asks for his father, but it is now more like he talks about him visiting him in his dreams. That works for both of us.

On July 10, 2011, Zach was hit by a car while crossing a crosswalk in an electric wheelchair. He had been living in a group home and getting ready to begin an internship with CNN Sports in Connecticut. I spoke to him on the phone while he was in the emergency room and he said he planned to come down to stay with Nate's Mom to recover, and we would go bowling. The next day I got a call from Nancy to let me know that he had passed away. He had been sent home and told to take Tylenol if he had any pain and to call them in the morning. I won't go into details, but he died in his sleep.

A few years later, Nate and his mom moved down to SC for financial reasons and spent several years there. I called Nate every day to talk to him and make sure he was doing ok. Nancy, said I only missed no more than six days. I also went down four times to spend time with them. Now they are back in Vermont, and we are working together again. He and Nancy have been such a strong influence and support in my life. Some have told me I have taken caregiving for him too far. Maybe, but I have become friends with one of the most amazing human beings on the planet. He has inspired me in so many ways, and if he can smile and laugh while being in his condition, he is my mentor.

RE-ENTRY AND BEYOND

In 1971, I had just returned to Washington DC from Brazil, where I had stayed for a 1+ year program with the International Farm Youth Exchange (now known as the International 4-H Youth Exchange or IFYE). I was on the Youth Development Program, which allowed me to do more community work and help set up programs in the community. On returning, I was asked to participate in a debriefing program. Besides myself, there were many people from all over the world. They had just finished a stay in the US representing their countries.

One day I was asked to go to the 4-H office and fill out some debriefing questionnaires. In the room there was a person from the Philippines. As we were sitting there filling out the forms, I noticed he was staring at me. Knowing I had to finish the questions, I kept writing. I looked up, and he was still looking my way. Suddenly he said, "What are you in for?" Not knowing what he meant I said, "Excuse me?" He replied, "What are you in for?" and then he laughed and introduced himself. "I am Jose Andre Sotto, from the Philippines. Who are you?" he said. I introduced myself, and we chatted for a while. We finished the questions and went down for a little lunch.

During that week I got to know him well, and we became great friends. When he went back to his country, we kept in touch through snail mail, which was the only way unless we used the phone, which was quite expensive for long distance. Now, this was during the Marcos Regime when there was a lot of turmoil in the Philippines, and the letters became less and less frequent. He never explained what was happening, but I never asked either. All I knew was what I saw on the news, and that Imelda Marcos had a lot of shoes.

In 1974, I received a letter from Jose-asking me to be his best man at his wedding. I said sure. I had been working as an area rep for a foreign exchange program called Youth for Understanding out of Ann Arbor, Michigan which was not too far from where Jose was to be married in Canada. Yes, Canada. He had moved there for reasons I am not sure about, but he was now living in Windsor, Ontario.

So, I took advantage of a business trip to Ann Arbor and added the wedding to the itinerary, which was to be the same week. I took a cab from Ann Arbor to Windsor which was not that far. When I got to the address, I got out of the cab and saw this short, smiling Philippine guy running toward me and knocking me over with all my luggage around me. It was so good to see him, as it had been several years. I asked him why he wanted me to be his best man and not someone closer to him. He simply stated that he did not know anyone else with such a passion for justice, compassion for all people, and a love for life than I had. He and I were very similar in so many ways but he was one of the most compassionate people I have ever known. Our relationship was mostly on paper through letters and stories, but when we physically met again for the first time since our days in Washington, it was like we were brothers. I have never been so proud to know someone like Jose.

One of the events we went to was a bowling night with the entire wedding party. As we had a bite to eat, the TV that was on nearby showed President Nixon speaking. Jose, having an interest in politics, turned up the volume. I did not know it then, but this would become one of the most famous speeches he would deliver. It was the night he resigned from office. Wow! I leave the country with one president in office, and I go back to the same country with a different president in office in less than a week. Now, for those of you who were not around then, this was when the Pentagon Papers, Watergate, and the Vietnam War were going on, and now more than 40 years later we see it crop up in the government during all this Muler investigation, impeachment talk and in movies like The Post. So, it was a very historic event I was witnessing with a friend, who was an amazing human being.

The wedding was wonderful, and we kept in touch for some time. Time passed, and we lost touch. He became very involved in the community and was quite famous, which I did not know. Shows how much you know someone, good or bad. This was good.

I received a letter asking me if I would go to Canada and meet my new godson-to-be. That was his way of asking me if I would be his son's godfather. I said yes, but when the time came I was not able to attend, because of something at work and I was devastated. He suggested I do it by proxy, so I agreed. I did not want to let him down. Time went on, and I found out JoJo was to be confirmed in the church. I had to do this one and gladly went, no matter what was going on. We hit it off and became close. We took pictures with my camera and went for walks with him on my shoulders. I kept in touch for a while and then, as usual, life happened. I remember sending a letter to him and my goddaughter GiGi, who was JoJo's cousin, stating that I felt so bad I had not fulfilled my commitment as a godfather. I mentioned that I had wished the position had come with a book of instructions.

Time passed and I tried several times to connect, but failed until I found Jose online. His profile came up as a minister in Canada. I let them know I would like to connect, but there was no response. I felt that the messages were not getting to him. One day I found JoJo, or Jonathan, on Facebook. I asked if this was the JoJo who had a godfather in the US. He responded with a big "Yes!" I told him I would like to meet up with him and his father. He agreed it would be a good thing.

After a while I got a message from JoJo. Jose had been ill and died. I was devastated, and because of the lack of time to get there, I would miss the funeral. JoJo was so kind and told me it was OK. He knew how special our friendship was, and life just happens. There were no ill feelings. My godson is now in his 30s, lives in Singapore and very successful I am so proud of him. I did not realize it until recently that JoJo was my Caregiver, in a sense. He let me know that I was ok and that whatever happened in the past is just the past. I should not feel any guilt, and he did not dislike me for any reason.

I told him one day, I should write a book on "How To Be A Godparent' or "How Not To Be A Godparent." Who knows?

I have been in touch with JoJo through Facebook. He sent me a video of him talking about his beliefs and feelings about a lot of things. A lot of it had to do with discrimination and injustice.

My response was as follows:

"Thank you, JoJo. I have lived all over the globe and have seen, in many forms, the homogenization of the races, religions, skin colors, and sexual orientations. Unfortunately, skin pigment is one of the easiest and most common to attack. The suppression of diversity has been around since the beginning of humanity. The superior race, society or religion, Americanizing the American Indians, African Slavery, Japanese segregation on the premise that they are a threat rather than American, the Jews in Germany, the Irish in NYC are sad comtntaries for the human race. Also the idea that Taiwan people are not a race by China and so many others are the crimes that have come out of the fight to be the superior race, religion or sex are still part of our dialogue today. My ignorance as a child and being sheltered in so many ways as a White American growing up in a white society that would not allow the image of a black person on the TV screen in a positive light, allowed me to question freely why they were treated like that."…"I had no concept of race, but it was the first time I became aware of the diversity of our world. From that point on I embraced diversity and questioned why discrimination made it OK to degrade others of a different race, creed or gender. Beauty pageants are also guilty of trying to homogenize and purify the female gender in the name of perfection.

This year I am preparing to adopt a young man who, for the past 25 years, since he was nine, I have considered my son. He is the polar opposite of me and only until recently have I heard the response when showing someone a picture of him, "Oh, he is Black" as if I didn't know. My response is usually, "Oh really? I hadn't noticed." I also have my two godchildren who are in Canada. When I show a picture of them, they say, "I thought they were Canadian." "JoJo and GiGi are Filipino Canadians." This leads me to believe we are stepping back, and that we are walking with eyes wide shut. Thank you, JoJo, for posting your video. I question the future with so many of the events that have happened in the last several years. Diversity is not alive and well these days. When I must explain and defend myself because of my beliefs, I fear we are on a long and winding road to a better world and one that is more accepting of the diverse nature of it. We are so connected in so many ways, and yet we are disconnected in so many other ways. I have faith that what I do will make a difference in whatever the world will be for my children, biological or not. I say we all need to be more diligent and aware of injustices like the one you presented in this post. To stay silent is only fuel for a status quo society. I love you JoJo and GiGi, and hope to see you face to face soon. Keep up the awareness."

So Long My Friend

Yanni has a CD out with a piece called "So Long My Friend" as one of the selections. I wasn't familiar with it until one day while staying with my friend Benjie, who Mark, and I met in Cancun. He played the song for me and thought, after reading the title, it would mean a lot to me. I immediately remembered the tune. Mark had heard it on TV or radio and had said he really liked it. It seemed special to him at the time, but I did not know why. Benjie gave me the name of the CD. I am fond of the work of Yanni. While I was there, I must have listened to it a dozen times. It was almost like I was trying to lock the tune into my memory. In time it would become part of my healing process. I almost felt that with this song, Mark was trying to say something, or just say good-bye. I played it so much that day Benjie threatened to take off the repeat button.

Since Mark's death, (and later on Burt, and so many others), I found that friends, my photography, writing, travel and music, are all part of the healing process. They are also part of growing. I learn more each day about myself, and that we all must work together to better understand all the pain and tragedy that accompanies AIDS, cancer, TBI, physical and mental disabilities, Alzheimer's, diabetes, and so many others.

Before Mark's illness had begun to advance into full-blown AIDS, his Aunt Barbara and I spoke on the phone many times. I had never met her, and yet I was talking to her as if I had known her for years. Her telling me that if I ever needed to vent she would be there for me, were reassuring to me. She also said it was important that I say what I have to say to him before anything serious happens that will make it impossible to do so, like Dementia, Alzheimer's, or death. I knew that was true from the death of my mom and partly from my father, but to think Mark would not be around or out of his senses didn't seem real yet, or I did not want to entertain that idea. Yet I knew I had to do it.

As a side note, I recently had a conversation with my son Homer about me not being here too much longer, and what he will have to do after I am gone. He said that he did not want to think about me not being here, yet he said he wanted to be complete as much as possible with me. Such a good boy he has turned out to be. I'm proud of him.

Mark and I had sessions at the house where we said what we thought needed to be said, but it never seemed to be complete for some reason. It was as if being complete was acknowledging that he might not make it. It was right around the time when we had a huge argument about leaving each other by death. It was ten years since the day that we became friends. I wanted to let him know how much our relationship meant and it was hard to verbalize it, so I wrote a letter in the form of a poem:

Ten years ago, the stage was set
In a place, in time where our paths had met
Like breadsticks, we stood, another face in the crowd
We knew where we stood and to our limits what we allowed.

I looked, you looked, as friends we became one
We allowed our friendship to grow
Now ten years have passed with the cycles of the sun
And yet there is still room to grow.

I know your pain
I cannot feel
I understand your joys
I cannot express

I know your recent tears, true and flowing
I cannot shed for you
But one thing I know, feel, experience and share
Is your love for life, true and giving, stern and honest

If that is all I have to show for these ten years as your friend
Then I am a wealthy man
I apologize not for any of the ten years
As each moment prepared me for the next, good and bad

I know your wishes for me are to be strong, well and organized
As miracles never cease
My wishes for you are simple and true
To accept the love being given to you and around
you with no pain and with much dignity

The gifts and flowers are only a symbol of
the caring we have for each other
The few days I spent with your Mom gave me new life
and hope and a chance to recall all that was good
With the years I spent with Mom and how they were so alike
With unconditional love for their children

I thank you for the chance to share these years
And I hope there will be more to come
But all in all, I am thankful for having you as
my friend I can truly say it has been fun

It was the true and fearful thought of the moments to come that gave me the courage and the chance to share them with him

From that moment on we made a point of continuing to work together as a team to make the last days the best. Many of Mark's friends were not sure about it, as they brought sadness and drama along for the ride. If we were angry, we shared it. We did this before, but it became mundane and routine. This time, it was out of urgency and purpose. If something good happened, we made it better. We laughed more than ever, and yet were not afraid to cry. We were taking the bull of reality by the horns and dealing with it the best way we knew how. Life in general had become so precious to us, as did our friends and relationships around us. There were times when it was hard to continue, but together as a team, we all benefited from it. People around us could see a positive change and liked it, and were willing to tell us they saw it.

Since then, I have tried to make each day special and take care of the things that need taken care of. In the hospital, the nurses couldn't believe Mark had such a good spirit. I am sure that it is hard knowing that your time is short. Being only 32, he must have felt cheated at times. I only hope I have that same strength when my time comes. There were also times when I could see him feeling guilty that his leaving was his fault, or that he had to take responsibility for it. Seeing his mother sad made it even harder. Yet, he would pull himself out of that emotion, and make a joke or change to a lighter subject.

He accepted death, and I welcomed it during the last few hours of his pain. Those last two days were the most intense when we had to say our last good-byes. We stayed up all night the night before he died. We talked about old times, and the days to come when I would need to be strong. It was hard to think we had shared so much and taken so much for granted. Talking that night washed any guilt away. His mom was sleeping in the other room. It gave us a good chance to be together for the last time. At times his hand shook. He would pass it off as a sharp pain, but I knew he was scared. He was about to do something we all will do and yet are never prepared for. He was about to die.

But what is death? Will we ever know? And should we know? I created a program called Legacy. I will explain most of it in another chapter, but basically, it deals with three questions that can give each of us the power to create our own legacy. I wished I had created this before I lost Mark, although I think he was well aware of the legacy he was leaving.

The night before he died, he wanted only his mom and me there. It was almost like he knew the time was near. The morphine they gave him was the strongest yet. Still, it wasn't enough to get rid of the pain.

The nurse had told me that if he had too much, his breathing would stop and there would be nothing anyone could do. I didn't want him to know, because I didn't want him to knowingly take too much.

It was about 6:30 AM when Mark asked me to get the nurse to give him another booster of morphine. The pain was so intense that the drug was useless. He was screaming when I went to the nurse and told her what he said. She looked at me as if to say, "You know what this could mean." I did not want him in any more pain than he could handle.

She came in and gave him the booster. For the next hour, he faded in and out of consciousness. I knew he was more comfortable. His mother stood on the right side of the bed, and I stood on the left. We held his hands and spoke to him to calm him while rubbing lotion on his arms and hands, letting him know we were still here. I remember his mother saying quietly to herself, "It isn't fair. It isn't fair; I'm supposed to go first."

My heart went out to her that morning. Yet, she was strong and she didn't let him see her pain. We talked to Mark throughout the hour. It was the longest hour I have ever spent, and I hope I never have to do it again. The morphine was working as the pain lessened, but he was fading slowly. His words were slurred. I mentioned to him that I thought he was on the best high he had ever been on. He smiled.

Just then he gasped for breath and held it, as if he were going underwater. Then, he let it out slowly and stopped breathing. I thought it was the end when out came another gasp and the words "Help me, help me, help me."

I felt helpless as I held his hand and talked to him. He then was able to say faintly, "I love you," and there were no more breaths, and he was still. We must have sat there for a minute, but it felt like forever. We were waiting for another breath that would never come. The nurse came and took his pulse. He died on July 31, 1992, at 7:31 AM. As I stood there, I thought about the day in Cancun when we sat at the water's edge and watched the sunset. I remembered how intense that moment was, and watching how slowly it sank in the horizon. While we were going through that last hour in the hospital the sun was rising, and just as he had sat still watching the sunset, he was still again as the morning sun lit up his face through the window.

His mom and I walked out of the room holding each other. We sat in the waiting room where we met his step-father and the minister. We were all like lost children in the woods with no clue how to get back.

That day was the day I had to take down my exhibition of photos, which gave me something to keep me busy. It gave me a chance to look at all my photographs in a new light. I had just lost my best friend and companion as he slipped away into the sunrise. Now I was ending another part of my life. The name of the show was "Faded Dreams, Broken Windows," which seemed more than appropriate. They were photos of abandoned houses and parts of structures that have been left by the wayside, and were once someone's dream house or pride and joy. As I took each picture down, I studied them in a way I had never seen them, and remembered when they were taken and what Mark and I were doing then.

Mark's death and the ordeal was a faded dream, and the things we couldn't finish were the broken windows. Windows to the future that were now broken or boarded up. How temporary we are here on this planet, yet we live life as if we were immortal. We judge, push and shove, forget and remember too late the good simple things, reality, and our existence.

In writing this book I have been attempting to fix the windows and take down the boards so that you and others might look through them and take from the experience Mark and I had. The growth I experienced as a Caregiver, and hopefully some of the strength I gained, can become visible to those who are looking for that strength that we all need as Caregivers and those who we care for.

You don't have to look any farther than your own windows that you may have already boarded up and locked. But if we could only put shutters or shades, we could spend less time boarding things up and more time in our gardens.

There is a video online that is a wonderful story called, "The Window" a Christmas story and there is another version not for Christmas. It shows how we all have a window to the world in our mine and can show others what we can see through that window. Quite inspiring.

https://www.youtube.com/watch?v=4WNWzvcA8yY

What I have learned is that if I just take some time each day and look at the good in it the days goes a bit smoother. If it is a bad day, I look at how that bad can be transformed to be manageable and more positive. When I have a dispute with someone, it is easier to confront it than wallow in it, letting it fester in my mind and making it worse than it is. It is also healthier to confront things as they come along and deal with them, because anger, sadness, and uneasiness can make us sick emotionally and physically. Take time to look at each day and make it the best day you can. Do something good for someone each day. We all want to make a difference in life. As history has proven, sometimes that difference can be negative. I aim to make a difference that is healthy and good. The phrase "You don't know what you have until it's gone." is so true. Don't wait until it is gone. Learn how to leave a legacy that you are proud of. Treat everyone the way you would want others to treat you. With respect and dignity.

JUST VENTING

A while ago a coworker asked me why I spent so many years taking care of Nate, and was I trying to prove something. Wow! At first I wanted to try to defend myself, but could not find the words through my anger. I probably would have said something I would have regretted. I walked away from the opportunity. That made me think a lot about why I did spend so many years with him. I kept trying to figure out what I was trying to prove, or if I was trying to prove anything. I began to realize that most of the people I had cared for, I did so to the end. Why? I could not say. Maybe it was just my nature.

I pondered and searched, and every time I came up with that self-centered approach to everything. Was I trying to prove that I was stronger or better than anyone else? The more I thought, the more I got angry with myself and the person who asked me the question.

Eventually, I tried to forget about it and just did what I normally do - give care. After taking a class in astrology and looking at all the charts and characteristics of who I was within the realm of astrology, I started to understand that it could be bigger than myself and all of us. I started to look at everyone differently, as we all have specific characteristics of who we are. The "Why?" question was still looming over me. I could not let it go. I had spent my whole life as a Caregiver of some sort and had no answers that would give self-satisfactory justification to the "Why's".

A few months went by, and I was asked almost the same question by a friend. This time I had pondered the question, and at least had something to say. I said, "Nathan had no control of who he was, how he got that way and had CP. He was lucky to have fallen into the hands of an amazing couple who were Caregivers in the strongest sense. Nate didn't get a day off from being who he was or having what he had. So, who am I to take time off if I am to call myself a Caregiver? One thing I noticed about people who needed to be cared for, having friends or people around them to stay with them for a long time is rare. Most of the people who called him a friend have not seen him in years and have no idea how much just having a friend can mean to the success of their living experience. When Nate moved to another town, I followed him. When he went to another state for several years, I called him every day, and when he came back, I spent four months working with him at night without pay as our system, as messed up as it is, states that you must have six months before services would kick in. He had no one but his mom, who was in her mid-seventies and several family members who looked in on them occasionally. He could not get into his wheelchair because his mom could not lift him and lying in bed all day, well, you try that, especially when you have no control of your limbs and neck muscles. His mom, members of his family, and myself were his only constants. That is why. He is a human being with needs that the system does not seem to understand, and to take care of the needs of someone like him is only a business to most. It is a paycheck, and something for the resume.

I feel he deserves some dignity and respect, and should have the right to be able to live a healthy life. Many of the people I knew in the early days were shoved into institutions and kept out of sight. Thank God that has changed. That 'we should hide them from society' attitude is still with us about homeless, drug addicts, mental health and so many others. I sometimes feel like we may be going back to that with some of the legislation I see coming down the road. To see people who have little voice or mobility being dragged out of the capital building and arrested for disturbing the peace makes me shudder. That is why I have stayed so long. Not for my ego, my glory, or feeling good, but for trying to do what is right, just, and fair. I am not saying there isn't a little ego in the mix. And yes, it does make me feel good when someone recognizes my work. But I have lived my whole life watching society put people down for their skin color, their beliefs, their disability, their sexual orientation or their gender (selected or natural). Our society has failed so many for being different for so long it has become just business as usual. Shame on us! How dare you ask me why or judge me for doing what is right and just in my mind and heart?"

After I was through, he just looked and said, "I think I touched a nerve." I said, "Yes you did, and I am so clear about the 'why's I have been wrestling with." And I am clear, crystal clear. It is not just people with disabilities that we can see, it is about the kids I have been fortunate enough to work with who were dealt a bad hand in life. Homer, who is now my son, was one of them. Many of my kids in school who I still am in contact with have been misunderstood in so many ways. We wonder how they turned out the way they did: arrogant, angry and confused. Some people yell at them and make them feel wrong at every turn. Parents, teachers, people in the community, and society in general have been stuck on this assumption that they are just bad kids. Many of the "bad kids" I worked with are living productive lives and were just in a system that didn't understand them, and they just did not fit in any of the boxes we had created for them. One of the biggest problems is that we tend to dictate or teach, but not listen. Granted, there are a lot of amazing programs that do wonderful things with the kids and are quite successful, but our educational system is archaic and well overdue for an overhaul, and I don't see that happening any time soon.

I know we have experimented with so many types of education, and some have worked and others not so much. This is difficult, as it costs money to do this and change gears midstream. Because taxes come from the public, the road is slow, yet people complain.

I am not trying to say that all is lost in the system; I am trying to shed light on the things that do not work well with some of our youth and all the other populations who have no voice. This has been true for many, many years. Remember the 60s, the hippy movement, and all the experimental drugs? Many of them were living the dream. They found a way to do it. Veterans who came back from the war in most wars were considered heroes, and then came Vietnam. Many of my friends and classmates went, and some came back broken and shoved aside. Remember "Midnight Cowboy" and "Forrest Gump"? We are able to use this tragedy to enhance our entertainment, and yet we still cannot see that it is not just a story or script in a movie. It is real. How many homeless people have you ever seen, and have you ever wondered what their life was like before this or how it happened? When I lived in NYC, I asked many of them how they ended up homeless. It is amazing the stories you will hear. You should try it. Sure, there are a lot of panhandlers who could do better, and are making more than me by being convincing and begging, but until we find out their story, who are we to judge?

I recently made a judgement about a woman I saw walking on the sidewalk with a baby in a stroller. She had a cigarette in one hand and her phone in the other pushing the stroller with her stomach. She was dressed in spikes and some flashy clothes. My comment was that I wonder how the kid was going to turn out. I posted it not thinking it would get attention. One of my students, Michael who used to help me with Burt, called me on it and said, "It is not your judgement that is important but what you do to make the change or how you help that counts." Way to go Michael. I taught you well.

I had a student who was a real hell-raiser. He was wiry and angry. He had been a hard kid to raise and it was just too much for the parents. His father's way of dealing with the situation was to tell him to get the hell out. His mom was using, and his brothers were off on their own. He had been staying with a relative, and it was too much for her at her age, so he was told to find someplace to live. He was 16, blamed for being who he was, and no one was taking responsibility for their actions and influence on him. I am not saying that he had no blame in this, but there must have been some underlying reason for his rebellion. Of course he was going to act out in school, because that was his way of getting someone to listen to him and see him. The old saying goes, "Any attention is good attention". I was assigned to him in school, along with several others like him. I had to sit with each one of them for a while to make sure they were okay, then had to go to the next.

They all looked forward to me being there as they could talk to me. I was later told that I was one of the only people in the school who could handle them without burning out and giving them detention every time they acted out. When I saw them ready to act out, I would say, "Let's go for a walk." Many times we would say nothing, but a lot of the time they would vent because I would listen without judgment.

One day he came into the office crying. He had no place to live. He planned on stealing a car and driving to another state and living in the woods where he could stay away from people. I tried to tell him that he needed to graduate, but he would not listen. I had just been offered a job in a non-profit for a lot more money, and told him to go to his aunt and beg her to let him stay with her until the end of the week. I told him I would let him stay in one of my rooms as I have a 16 room Victorian. He agreed, and I told him we would work out the details. I had only four rules. He had to stay in school, look for a job, no drugs in the house, and he had to graduate. If he did not graduate in June then he would have to look for another place, but he was in control and responsible. So, from January to June he was my boarder. I gave him a chance to succeed, and he could not blame anyone else if he failed.

Most of my co-workers said I was crazy, and maybe I was, but he was a good kid. In the end, he abused his stay by selling drugs from the house, did not finish school, and never got a job. Yet I did not give up. We had many talks, and he knew how much it was hurting me. I am still in touch with him. He has a job, a girlfriend, and he graduated, but still has a way to go. But you know, every time I need help at the house, he is there. He takes me out to lunch and has paid me back some of what he owes me. He also remembers my birthday. It's a start. Now, what if I had given up? I was one of the only constants in his life, although he has now reunited with his family and has an entirely new vision of who they are and who he is with them. I am sure there will be some ups and downs and hiccups in the future, but they will be his ups and downs and hiccups.

What I am trying to convey is that we all have a responsibility as a Caregiver, whether it is as a parent, teacher, relative, community member or law enforcement to stick with the children we are bringing into this world, even though their generation is wired to the internet. We must understand why they are the way they are and not judge them by our experience of growing up. Look back to when you were growing up. It was so different than your parents' upbringing, yet they most likely were there when you needed them, and you turned out ok. It has been like this for as long as society has existed. Our minds and eyes need to be more open.

On the flip side, many kids who are grown-ups are now judging their elderly parents for what they did, as now it goes both ways when the child becomes the Caregiver of the parents. They should never be thought of as a burden. When the time comes, you will need dignity and respect from the younger generation.

The Lion King had it right. "The Circle of Life" by Elton John. Listen to the words and see what you think. Live on the kinder side of life. Take time to think about who you are judging, before you speak. Look at how wonderful the world is and can be. Be the change you want to see. The phrase "Life sucks" is a common judgment when we are unhappy with something. Life does not suck. Life is amazing and miraculous. What people do to themselves and others sucks. We have created the suck in life. So, let's create a wonderful life instead. Think before you do something. It is easy to give someone the finger. I did it just this evening when someone was behind me with their high beams on and was tailing me on the highway. When they passed me as I slowed down, I gave them the finger. The problem is that the only person who benefited from that finger was me. It made me angry, and I felt good by reacting the way I did. They just went on their merry way. It was all about me.

I hope you see what I am ranting about. If you do, tell me. I am more confused than I was before. But, thank you for putting up with me.

WHERE HAVE
ALL THE FLOWERS GONE

Being a Caregiver, support person, and a PCA, I have had to learn a lot about protocol, procedures, and just moral values, along with common sense. One of the programs I began to work as a peer educator for was the Harm Reduction Program called "The Sharing Community". It was started in Yonkers by Rev. S. Burtner Ulrich and Rev. John P. Duffell. This program was created in the 70s, to ease the pressure on the community from the rapid influx of homelessness and substance abuse on the streets. St. John's Episcopal Church was opened to those who were on the streets to sleep and get a good breakfast. Many of the parishioners from both the Catholic and Episcopal congregations helped in any way they could.

From those meager beginnings, it has turned into one of the largest umbrella programs serving many homeless families and individuals, substance users, people with HIV, and people with many other mental health issues. It has become a multimillion-dollar program with many housing units for people who need it. It also deals with political issues at times, such as getting the word out about HIV and AIDS when it was so controversial. Being a part of this organization has opened many doors for me. It has especially raised my awareness of the issue of confidentiality. How do I talk about what is going on when I can't reference my findings? Sounds confusing? It is!

Within the realm of confidentiality, I have rediscovered many things within myself which I have to confront each day, especially as I get older. It wasn't until I was at one of the other jobs and someone asked me if it was true what they had heard about me. A breach of confidentiality and the creation of a rumor had occurred. I was the victim. It was like I had learned as much about the subject for occupational purposes as I could and now I was being tested. I was working with the program dealing with HIV, and someone assumed I was positive. This was when I realized how dangerous confidentiality could be in the wrong hands. Today with all the hacking of computers and the selling of information about us and what we do by companies we are supposed to trust, confidentiality is lost in the shuffle.

That incident opened a truckload of feelings and emotions that I am sure will not go away soon. As important as confidentiality is, it was also holding many issues back from progressing to the point where the public may not have begun to realize how devastating AIDS was, how prevalent it was and how vulnerable we all were. We think, "It can't happen to us." We had made it so hard for people to go out and get help because of the stigma and public opinion on the issue of AIDS.

I was in a support group where I met people still saying, they were afraid to talk to anyone about their loss or situation. It was there that became more aware of the sensitivity of confidentiality. "They wouldn't understand" or "What will they say if I discuss my situation with them?" or "What will they think of me?" We were dealing with an illness that, like cancer in the early years, leads a stigmatized existence where it is unsafe to talk to anyone known to have the disease, or someone related to one who had it. Cancer and many other illnesses was called consumption, and was believed to be transmitted through the air at one time.

I live in Vermont now and stigmas still exist with regards to race, sexuality, transgender and gay lifestyles, as well as with mental illness. Many people with disabilities become invisible. I take Nate out to the store and he will say hi to everyone he can. Most people say nothing. When someone does say hi back to him, I tell them they won the grand prize and that usually sparks a conversation. Some individuals are forced to hide and live a secret life if they are part of any of these groups.

The less we talk about and discuss these issues, the less we get done. It used to be, if you had the virus and were covered by insurance, there was no guarantee that you would not be dropped. If you took it to court, which took forever to go through, and had a lawyer who knew his or her stuff, you may or may not outlive the case such as in the movie Philadelphia, from 1993. Precious time was lost then and now. Most of us couldn't put a face on the virus until it hit home. Then it became a game of catch up to get as much information as possible and keep it to yourself. What would the neighbors say? This is also true for families with a relative who might be homeless, gay, transgender or on drugs.

We still have a large population who think it can't happen to them, either becoming infected or affected, and that includes all STDs. Many still look at the virus as contagious in ways that are not realistic. There is now a lot of literature out there which is so easy to acquire, as it is on the internet also on the internet. Most of it is free. Yet we tell ourselves, it can't happen to us. This is the consensus with most young people which means the use of condoms may go by the wayside. Many students have told me that it was something that only happened in the 80s and 90s.

For so many years, I would meet people who have joined the ranks in either category, affected or infected. Even today we still have the old fears, some of which are well-founded as I have found. But for the most part, they are just fears based on our ignorance. Everyone has been ignorant of everything at some point in their lives. We all have had to learn everything we know. Yet for some strange reason, even with our fears, we are not willing to learn the facts. It is a sad commentary about the human condition, but it is true.

When Mark was diagnosed, I experienced many of the same fears based on my ignorance, and I scrambled to learn everything I could about the issues. The more I spoke to people about it, the more I learned that there were people out there who cared and had compassion for Mark, and for myself as his Caregiver and friend. Of course, there were those who were cynical and rude, but for the most part, people were caring.

As I went along this journey, I closed the door to many things. It seemed more important that I take care of the things at hand. For a while, I would go out and make it a campaign to share as much information as I could. I would take any chance to talk about injustice and social discrimination, in all aspects of life. When you are in the center of it all, it is hard to stop the train and look at the scenery. We become engulfed with what needs to be done at that moment.

The few times I tried to get off the train on this caregiving journey I found when I got back, there was so much to catch up with and do. Feelings of abandonment, guilt, and sorrow came up from the one being cared for. These feelings were so strong that it was hard to retake those side trips. I began to understand why people would stay quiet about issues and just attend to the task at hand. Unless you are with someone who truly understands and are open to the fact that you are also affected deeply by the virus, taking these side-trips is not wise. I would find myself sometimes in the shoulda, woulda, coulda corner. I should have stayed with him. I could have left my own wellness on the sideline, and I would have been more conscious of his or her feelings if I had paid more attention. What a disappointment it was when I thought I did something good and then felt I might be wrong. It can become debilitating. I had to either learn how to pick up my feelings and deal with them later, or discuss them ASAP. Mark and I were lucky. We were able to resolve this, so we were both comfortable before it was too late. When Mark wasn't showing signs of the illness, it was like we had just won the lottery. We were planting new positive seeds in our garden that we thought would carry us through to the end, whenever that would be. We were learning new ways of looking at the simple things in life. It was like that wonderful feeling when you enter a greenhouse full of flowers in the middle of winter. There was hope for a new spring. Life was a hoot, even with the knowledge that there may not be as much time left as we had thought. The walks in the park were special. Talking to each other was special. Remembering old times was special. Knowing that we were still alive and that we were making the best of it was special.

Suddenly, some of the flowers began to fade in this garden of the mind and spirit. More and new medications were the talk of the day. When do we bring in the wheelchair and the hospital bed? How long will he be able to go to work? What does it take to prove to Social Security Disability that he is ill and unable to function at work? Should we change our eating habits? Will we be able to pay the bills?

All that seemed to be left in the garden was the greenery. The only flowers were cut flowers on the nightstand next to the hospital bed. How do we get the flowers back? Where have they all gone?

At that point, I realized that the sad thing was that the flowers were all still there. We just needed to water them and try even harder to keep them alive. I spoke to Mark and told him that I felt it isn't over yet. He was still alive, breathing, laughing, and of sound mind. We should be thankful for that. The idea of appreciating the little things was still real.

One evening we invited some of his friends over. These were the same friends Mark didn't want to see because he was so ill. He didn't want them to see him like this. Those friends stayed with him to the end. In the hospital, his spirit was one of jokes and making new memories for those he would be leaving behind. Somehow, I think he knew exactly what he was doing all the way. Recently I heard the phrase, Team Derek, or Team Cynthia which refers to the people who make up their support system. It is the same thing we were doing then but with a different name attached.

That evening I saw someone with more courage and compassion than I have ever seen and may ever see again in one person. Sure, there were times when the journey made some unscheduled stops that made it hard to stay conscious of where and who we were. It was still a lesson I will carry with me forever. A lesson I pray I never lose sight of.

While he was in the hospital, there were times when he had twenty people in his room. He was "entertaining the troops," he said. One of those days was extra special and gave him a chance to give back a little. A group of musicians and singers called "Celebration" from Old Greenwich, Connecticut, was in the hospital. They would go around, room by room, and entertain the patients. They asked him if he had any requests and he gave them three. These three songs were songs that meant more than anything to him.

When he was younger he used to listen to Joe Cocker sing, "With a Little Help from My Friends." That song was the essence of who Mark was. The second song he had them sing was "You Got a Friend" by James Taylor. He wanted his friends to know how he felt about them and how special they were. The third was from the musical Cats called "Memories". That was the first Broadway Show we had seen together. That song meant so much to him and was like he was saying, "Thanks for the memories."

He was trying to create a bouquet for us to take with us on our journeys. That day we knew that the flowers were still there all along. They were fed by Mark's love. We just had to believe they were there and receive them.

THE HEART OF YONKERS

1992 was a year that many changes occurred in my life, with the death of my Dad, Mark, and Elsie. I wa involved with a support group for people who had lost someone with AIDS and it was truly an eye-opener in so many ways. Moving on was a challenge guilt set in when I was going through clothes, books, and other items of theirs that I had to let go of, and yet I wanted to keep everything. I had to start dealing with Mark's stuff by letting go of something that meant a lot to both of us. I put some of Mark's clothes that I had bought him when he could not go out, in a box, and took them to the Salvation Army. I could not have known how hard that would be. However, it helped jump start things I had to do, and I was able to move on to pick and choose what I would keep and let go of. I still have some things of both my Dad's and Mark's, but they are things that were symbolic of their love and commitment.

Searching for a new direction or purpose in life, I was grasping at straws at times. I wanted to move on to new adventures, but felt so alone. It was tough to realize how much I depended on Mark and how much he depended on me. I had a new roommate, but it was not the same. I knew I had to move to another apartment, as keeping up with the rent and the expenses would get more and more difficult, so I looked for another place in Stamford. There were a lot of low-income buildings and apartments that would be affordable. I finally found a place not too far away that was nice, and I would be the only tenant. It was a house with a back yard and garage. It was a great deal for the price, so I took it.

As a photographer, I was working in a lot of venues and I needed an agent or someone who could guide me through the things I had to do to succeed at what I love to do. I was on the board of the Stamford Art Society and was able to secure several one-person shows. That gave me some exposure, and I was able to network very well. I was still in mourning over Mark's death, and quite exhausted. I met a minister in Old Greenwich, CT who had connections to the HIV/AIDS community. He knew someone who was good at marketing, and said he needed help and felt I had a lot to offer.

When we met, I found a strong, brilliant, powerful individual who had quite a history with the international media, major ground-breaking entertainment and gave me so much help. He was good at pushing me to do better and keep moving. I did have little handyman jobs all over Greenwich and Stamford, and they did pay well, but my first love was photography. One of the events I attended was a showing of a movie called, "One Foot on a Banana Peel, One Foot in the Grave" produced by Johnathan Demi. We were to meet him for some award of sorts. The evening went well, and the movie was powerful. It was about the daily lives of people with HIV through their eyes. As he went to look for Mr. Demi, I went to the coat line. I was in awe of how many familiar faces in the film industry were there and was so distracted that when I turned around, I bumped into a minister and knocked him over. After helping him up, we introduced ourselves. His name was Rev. S. Burtner Ulrich, and had a parish in Yonkers. We chatted for a while and he eventually gave me his card.

I had no idea how much he would be a factor in changing the direction of my life. He needed a photographer for his project to restore some of the windows in his church, which dated back to the 1600s and was about to celebrate its 300th year in Yonkers. I was interested and followed up with a meeting at the church a few weeks later.

Burt was well known in Yonkers, and when he was about to retire, one of the headlines about him in the papers was "The Heart of Yonkers," and the street was named after him where the church was located. His influence in that area went as far back as the late 60s. My first meeting was soon after our meeting at the movie showing, and he gave me a tour of the church. It was quite a relic of a church, and so much history attached to it. In the weeks after, I took many shots of the windows and the church. The natural lighting was interesting. It seemed to have a mystical feeling to it, but very solemn in a wonderful way. My first meeting with the parish to show my photos was with the Women's Guild. When I arrived, I had jeans and a t-shirt, as I had just come from a landscaping job. I brought clothes to change into, but I must have been a sight. One of the women would not let me in, as I looked like one of the many homeless guys who would ask for money from Fr. Burt. I knocked again, and she said he was busy and shut the door. It reminded me of the scene in the movie, "The Wizard of Oz" where the doorman would not let them in to see the Wizard. I waited a while outside until I saw Fr. Burt in the hall. He let me in, and I told him what had happened. He laughed and told me to go and change and clean up, and meet him in the meeting room.

Once I had changed, I came into the meeting room and sat next to Fr. Burt. The woman who told me to go away was sitting right in front of me, confused and embarrassed. Finally, Fr. Burt introduced me, and I proceeded to show the slides of their beautiful windows. It went well, and the woman came up to me and apologized profusely. I let her know it was all right.

After a while, I became a familiar face around the church, and Burt had introduced me to the program partly housed in the church facilities called The Sharing Community. I told Burt I had just lost Mark to AIDS, and he said that he had an extensive program for HIV/AIDS, homelessness, and substance abuse. He told me to meet with the director and see if he could use me. The meeting went well, and he told me he was looking for someone to head the peer education program they had established for HIV/AIDS and substance abuse. I told him I would think about it.

It did not take long for me to decide as I wanted to help with the education of this virus in the community, and especially in the schools. So I accepted, and I was on my way to beginning another incredible journey. I was free to get involved in all aspects of the programs and create new ones that would be geared to educating the community. I formed a peer education group comprised of people who were HIV positive, and many were connected to the substance abuse programs. I even had a group of teens who were willing to learn as much about the virus and substance abuse as they could and go into the schools to discuss the issues with their peers. It was very successful as a peer program, and at the time it was one of the only ones in Yonkers.

One of the issues I was confronted with, especially with the adults in the group who was HIV positive, was that they were afraid they would not be able to leave any legacy to their children and friends. We all need to make a difference in life while we are here and alive. This was something I found prevalent with people who felt they had very little time left, as at that time the virus was a death sentence. I spent a lot of time studying the idea of legacy, and after many months of research I created a program called "Legacy." My caregiving skills were in full gear. It was a little different than caring for one individual, but many of the components were the same. For instance, I had to find out what the needs of my group and the individuals in it were so I could address them in the best way I could. Taking care of some of their needs and elaborating on them in group sessions was vital. I had to understand and adapt myself to their lifestyle and their issues, which were so different from mine that I had to put myself in their shoes some days. We were a close-knit group, and many of them had been homeless and were part of the substance abuse crowd in the area. In many ways, they became my teachers and mentors to make this program work. And it did work. It worked very well.

Having this job gave me access to so many other venues in the HIV/AIDS community. Volunteers of America had a wonderful group who worked mainly on the education and exposure of the issues, as well as the caregiving aspects. We had workshops sponsored by the Ryan White Foundation's funding. Family Services of Westchester was one of the strongest supporters of these workshops. They were also the driving force in founding Camp VIVA.

Because I was a photographer, Burt asked me if I could take some photos of the programs. I became the go-to person with photography for many of the agencies. One day I was speaking to a person in my Legacy group. They asked me if there were venues to do some writing to leave their stories. I said I would check, but I did not think there were. I looked around, but there were only a few finished books and no ongoing venues to speak of. I decided to use my photography and their stories in an exhibit that eventually was shown in the Cathedral of St John the Divine. The name of the exhibit was, "If I Die Before I Wake," the same as this book, in memory of Mark, who used that phrase many times. I would take pictures of the person who was HIV positive, and they would write their stories in one or two-pages. It was very well attended by people from all over the world, and I could not have been luckier to have met Burt, who was on one of the committees at the Cathedral and knew many people there who allowed me to show my work. Eventually, the problem came when many of the people I photographed who signed a release died. Their families may not have known they had done this as there was such a negative stigma around AIDS, and especially in the black community. I received some letters from the mothers and families asking if I would please take these pictures down of their loved ones. They were all afraid of community retribution. I did not want to cause any pain for the families, so I agreed to take them down. This left me with the guilt of not following the wishes of the individual, but to harm a family was not my intention either. So, after three years of showing the exhibit all over the state of NY, I did not have enough pictures and scripts to continue, and it was time to move on to another project.

Being a Caregiver means that you are not only caring for one person, but that you have to also be concerned with their whole family and many of their friends. It proves that when one is ill, we are all affected. It is like a cluster bomb that hits us, one mother told me. My dreams of a book comprised of the photos and scripts in the exhibit were gone, and I had to protect the families and respect their wishes even though I had a signed release. The individuals had never consulted their families, and even though they had a right to do this on their own, I had to do damage control and prevent any more ill feelings. Just writing about this alone is enough. I do have some of the scripts that I will share anonymously at the end of this book.

As time went on, Burt and I became great friends, and quite a team. He had a place for me to stay in the rectory, which was an amazing piece of architecture. It had fireplaces in every room and had a grand staircase in the front and a tower which housed the spiral staircase the servants used to use in its hay day. My stay there was wonderful, and I was able to share the celebrations that were held there by the parish.

As an employee of The Sharing Community, I was asked to be their Santa. The church and The Sharing Community had a tradition of serving the homeless and anyone else who felt they needed a meal on Thanksgiving and Christmas. At last count when I was there, they had served 900 people. They were also allowed to take a meal home with them, and at Christmas they also got a gift. This was quite an undertaking. I was working for the Upper Room, which was part of the program that also worked with families affected by HIV, and they needed a Santa. So, I got dressed, and there I was - the best Santa ever. I enjoyed it, and would love doing it again.

As Santa, I would have the kids tell me what they wanted for Christmas. Most of these families had no money, food, or means to grant the wishes of their kids. I felt so bad and could not commit to their wishes, and said that Santa was also strapped for money this year but would do the best he could. It was criminal to me. One of the kids, Homer, had asked me if I was real and wanted to pull my beard. I told him if he did, it would not help him get the presents. He tried but for some reason, it got stuck on my lip and I yelled so he thought it was real. I did not know it then, but that young boy would become my son later in life and has been the challenge and joy of my life.

Fr. Burt had a house in Vermont where his dad lived, and we would go up some weekends and spend time working on the farm and house, as his dad was bed bound. His dad was an amazingly strong soul. He had polio and had problems walking most of his life. His love for gardening was not diminished by his disability, as he devised a way to do the weeding and planting. He used a piece of wood and put wheels on it. He would lie on his stomach and pull himself along in the garden with his tools and weed. He was well known for this in a small town in Vermont where he lived. I was truly amazed at his stamina. When his dad died, it was hard on Burt. He wanted to keep the house for his retirement, yet could not afford to keep it up while living in Yonkers.

I had just finished a program where I had worked with about 20 kids who were HIV positive, had been using drugs, and at one time were homeless. It was a small program, sort of a trial or experimental effort. In exchange for housing with family members if they needed it, food, and some healthcare, their job was to learn as much about HIV, homelessness and substance abuse as they could and go into the schools to talk to the students in the local schools. My job was to go to the churches where the sessions would take place and work with them. By the second year, not counting the ones who left early, I had been to at least 10 funerals and was at their deathbed for most of them. Because of the short success of the program, the individuals who funded it were not willing to be associated with it as in their eyes, it was not a success. The pilot program ended. It was a huge success, as it gave the kids a purpose for a while, and they changed the minds of many in the schools. I would have loved to have created one in a well-funded and substantial program because I could see great value in it. The hardest part was watching them get weaker and sicker in the end.

Not feeling good, I decided to get out of the programs I had been associated with at the church. I did not know it then, but burnout became the cause of my depression. One night I was sitting with Burt, and I just felt bad. I had pains in my chest, and my face felt cold and flushed at the same time. I drove myself to the hospital. They rushed me into the cardiac unit, and I was kept there for a week. Burt, who was home, felt ill and was rushed to the hospital. He too had suffered a cardiac episode.

By this time, Homer, the kid who sat on Santa's lap, was now living at the rectory. He was a handful, but he was amazing. I called him and told him that Burt and I were in the hospital. He hated hospitals and was not one to visit. I told him that when we got out, we were going to Vermont to recuperate for at least a month. He said he wanted to go, so we made arrangements for him to be up there for the summer.

We all stayed until Burt had to leave in September. He had been talking about what he was going to do with the house in Vermont he bought for his parents. The house was a three-story, one hundred and fifty-year-old farmhouse, six-plus acres, and had a year-round greenhouse that was a great place to have a Christmas party. I had no job to go back to, so we made arrangements for me to stay there and look for work. We made a deal. If I were to stay there and work on the house and make it a great place for a retirement home for him, I could stay there rent-free. "Done," I said. Little did I know how much work it would be.

So from 1997 to 2006 I remodeled the house and turned it into a great place to retire. Just before Burt retired, he developed diverticulitis and had much of his intestine removed. Eventually, he did retire and moved to Vermont. Even though it was a good decision health wise it was difficult as he was Chairman of the Board of St John's Hospital in Yonkers and would be assured the best care. After he arrived he got better and began his retirement.

The good times did not last long. Six months later he became ill and had a hard time walking. I was working two jobs and became his live-in Caregiver at night. This was the end of 2006, and he was dealing with the advanced stages of diabetes. He got worse, first losing one leg and a year later the other. The caregiving process was a bit more intense this time. He would wake up thinking that he had legs and get out of bed. Many times I found him on the floor with his head down and arm on the railing. Eventually, I decided to put the recliner next to the bed, and if he fell out even with the railings up, he would land on me or the recliner. That did not happen, but to this day I cannot sleep in a bed. I am working on it.

One day I was at home most of the afternoon, and was having a great conversation with Burt. We were talking about the weather, what was happening in town, and how the rectory had changed, which gave me a clue that he was not in Vermont at the moment, mentally. After we stopped talking, he asked me where Eli was. I said, "I am Eli." He said, "No, my Eli." I said, "Hold on, I'll go see." I went into the kitchen and did some dishes. I went back into the room a bit later where he was and said, "I heard you were looking for me."

He said, "Yeah, where were you?" I told him I was washing dishes. I asked him who that guy was he was talking to. He said, "I don't know, but he was a nice guy." That whole experience blew me away. It was the first sign of dementia. At least I know that the other guy who I am is a nice guy.

At the school where I worked, I'd had a student who graduated and was now married, but we were and still are best friends. Mike volunteered to come to the house at night while I was at work and sit with Burt and talk God stuff, as he was also very religious. It worked for me, and I cannot thank Michael White enough, (yes, my former student Michael) for his support, even up to the point where I cut off my finger and was flown down to Dartmouth with no one to bring me home since Burt was disabled. I called Mike, and even though he'd had a few beers, he came down and drove me to my car. I am so lucky to have so many students like Mike who have been there for me. I was on the receiving end of caregiving, and it was, I admit, uncomfortable. But it was well appreciated.

In 2008 I suffered a mild stroke. I woke up with one side of my body numb and thought I had just slept on the wrong side too long. So, I rolled over and fell back to sleep. When I woke up again, I tried to get out of bed and fell flat on the floor. I knew I could not expect Burt to help me, as he only had one leg. So, I crawled to the stairs and slid down to get dressed and hobbled to the car. I drove to the hospital with my left hand and left foot. I have never been so scared, but when I was brought home, I had to fend for myself pretty much, so the caregiving experience with Burt was about to turn into one hand washes the other deal. It was an eye-opening moment in my life. I did not know if I would get back full function of my arm and leg, and my face was sad on one side and all smiles on the other. My students would make fun of me at school when I was allowed to go back, as I had a distinctive step and slide walk. The kids used to like to follow me in a group and mimic my walk, thinking they were putting one over on me. One day, while walking down the hall, I could hear the group step-slide behind me. I turned around and told them they were not doing it right, and some of the kids were embarrassed that they got caught, but I told them if they were going to do it they needed to do it correctly. I showed them, and at least 15 kids followed behind me, mimicking me to the beat of my step, slide, and step. I endured the name Igor and others, but I told them that as long as they did it in fun and I was in on it, it was ok. One of the teachers saw it and could not stop laughing. I told her I was teaching them how to handle life with a stroke, along with a sense of humor.

As time went by, Burt got worse and worse, but we had so much support from this small community. It was amazing. I am very proud of the groups of supporters, from the churches to the hospital associations in Randolph, VT for the generous assistance and education they gave me. At Gifford Hospital, my doctors and Burt's doctors (who were sometimes the same) were amazing. I cannot thank them enough.

On October 5, 2012, I decided to go into work late, as Burt was not doing well, I had not slept, and the visiting nurses were coming in to work with us. I had been talking to Burt and had just cleaned his bed. We had been joking about a lot of things, and I knew he was in a different mood mentally. He was surely not in this time or reality. He believed he was still in Yonkers, and had to get his vestments ready for a wedding. I got up and spoke to the nurse for several minutes and glanced over to Burt. He seemed so peaceful, so I continued talking. I glanced over again and realized he had not moved, and looked *too* peaceful. I asked the other nurse to check him and see if he was OK. She did, but he had no pulse. Time stopped and all of a sudden. I did not know what to do. As a Caregiver, I was always in control and knew exactly what to do. This time, I was lost. I was not his Caregiver anymore. It was in the hands of others. Imagine yourself, living in your house, and the electricity goes out. The space you are in is being taken over by others, and the furniture is being moved. Someone comes in and cleans the floor and takes the furniture apart, and you just stand there. All this happened in several hours, and yet it felt like an instant.

I was told to call the coroner and the minister. I couldn't speak, so the nurse helped me. Here I was, a veteran Caregiver who had weathered Mark's death, Dad's death, and the deaths of so many others, and I was helpless. I have to say I now appreciate any and every nurse who exists on this planet, as they handled me (who was a basket case) with grace, charm, and dignity. My friend and neighbor, Tina Illsley and Veronica, a school associate, took me outside and hung with me. If it were not for them, I would not have made it. "The Heart of Yonkers" had just died, and they had no clue what that meant. Here, a great man who had changed the world and became the change he sought to see, had known people who were on the lowest rung of the ladder of life and treated them as he did the people who were high on the ladder - Bishops, royalty, powerful people and everything in between. He treated every person he met with the dignity and poise we should all aspire to. Now, he was being carried down the front stairs in a white body bag, and placed in the coroner's wagon.

Homer came up and stayed with me. Burt and I were the only true mentors he had known outside of a few mentors in the community who were connected with the school. The funeral was wonderful, and Homer walked behind the bagpipes with Burt's ashes, the hardest thing he had ever done. The bagpipes were played by Burt's friend, Steve Eubanks. Steve came to the house each week and talked "God Talk" as I would lovingly call it. It was a true gesture of the love Steve and Homer had for Burt. Of all the people I have met in my caregiving journey, Burt was the most humble, grand, gracious, spirited and spiritual, caring, just, compassionate and grateful people I have ever met. If I had to write another book, it would be about this amazing soul Burt, just so you might have the opportunity to meet "The Heart of Yonkers."

Thank Fullness

This essay was a submission to an art magazine for a program called Washington County Mental Health at The Learning Network in Vermont. The magazine is called Shock Wave, and it highlights the art and poetry of many individuals with diverse abilities.

At this stage in my life, now turning 70, I have had much to be thankful for. Having lived through some of the most turbulent, radical, and changing times ever, I have had much to ponder about how thankfulness fits into my life. I am first thankful for the words my grandfather said to me when I was a curious, confused and unstoppable teenager with an unsettling eye for injustice and ADD, which no one had discovered until long after the 60s. I was just a distractible young man who had a lot going on that was all positive. My grandfather said to me one day when I had to make a crucial decision, "If you are faced with a challenge or opportunity, look at it, study it well, chew it up and spit it out so to speak. If it still looks like something you could do, choose to do it. If you do it, you will know if you will succeed or not. If you don't do it, you will never know how great or not so great things could have come out of it."

I have lived my whole life doing just this. I have found that it has helped me to be thankful for the successes in my life, but more importantly, it has shown me how to be thankful for the tragedies in my life and the world, as many successes have been born from the tragedies I have witnessed and experienced. It all boils down to taking that leap of faith and making choices, but also knowing how to react to the results and to make the tragedies a more positive thing.

Working with the HIV population in the 80s and 90s, I witnessed a lot of death and personal loss. Yet I became aware that the people who were dying were giving me a gift for choosing to care for them and witness their passing away. It made me realize that there are two miraculous events in life we know little to nothing about besides life itself. Before life, and after life. These people let me witness a moment of transition in their existence that to me, to this day, leaves me in awe and in a calm that is like no other. It was that peaceful transition from life to another plane, if you believe that, or from life to non-life simply put, that opened my eyes to something greater than all of us. I met my son when he was nine, while his mom was in transition. His mom died of complications due to AIDS, and gave him that same gift. I now have a wonderful son who has shown me the beauty of a father-son relationship.

I am thankful for the choice I made to work in the institutions or "human warehouses" of the 60s, where people who were not "fitting into our social norms of abilities" were housed. It has given me something to compare my work with people who have different abilities, and to be aware that this could happen again given the changing winds of life.

I am thankful for having chosen to work with young people in the community, who for no fault of their own were brought into a situation that will stay with them for the rest of their lives. Their spunk, knowledge, and ambition, despite their adversity has given me a chance to realize what an amazing world we live in, and how we choose to lessen that amazingness in so many ways, yet we can change.

I am most thankful for having chosen to treat everyone I meet, from those full of life to the dying, from young to old, from homeless to the celebrities I have met in my life, with dignity and a non-judgmental approach as it has allowed me to see the inner glow deep inside every one of them.

Life has two sides to it. Good vs. evil. Calm vs. pain. Light vs. dark. Happy vs. sad. I choose the first of each of these, but am grateful for the ability to change a negative to a positive.

I finally appreciate the fullness of thanks.

Thank you.

Eli Shaw

INDEPENDENCE

Wars have been waged and fought. Men, women, and children have died, and borders have been redrawn for this thing called independence. We are all born without it and must learn and struggle for it until we are "of age" and then we start the cycle over after our parents cut the strings.

My work with people in wheelchairs has opened my eyes to this independence thing. We want to help, and yet by assisting we can delay the growth and success of this person being independant and living an independent existence. I know it is natural to want to help, but if you just ask first, that is a way that the Caregiver can begin being successful at giving care.

Independence is a learned privilege. It can be as simple as a feeling of freedom to do what we please. There are always laws and restrictions we encounter to control the masses. In some cultures, the laws are so restricting they attain the level of debilitation and death. Nazi Germany and North Korea are two examples of extreme lack of independence.

We here in the United States are lucky enough to live in a society where we are free to express, speak and do what we feel if it does not injure or attack the freedom of others. However. we had slavery, immigration issues, and religious persecution in some situations yet we live in the most unrestricted culture in the world along with several other countries that have reached a level of civility that allows acceptance of all.

Caregiving is an experience that is filled with cultural, human, natural and self restrictions. As a Caregiver for many years, I found my freedom to move freely or make decisions that are restricting, coupled with the demands and needs of another person.

As someone being cared for, restrictions are physical, mental, medical, environmental, and self-imposed. The self-imposed are the most difficult. We all have experienced someone saying "Let me help you," and then letting them. You know you can do it yourself, but it feels good to be waited on. The problem comes when we allow it to happen over and over. This is when we get lazy or too permissive to say no.

I have been in many situations where I am working with a teen or someone older who has not been given choices, or they have been told they couldn't succeed and feel worthless or would not amount to anything. They have learned to believe their critics, whether it be parents, teachers or even peers, and begin to believe what they are saying. They take on the belief that they are worthless. People who hold prisoners of war, the Nazis who detained the Jews, interrogation and detainment facilities use this method of mental and emotional deprivation to break down the will of the captive person.

This is when they look for comfort and acceptance from others, and many times for young people in our society it will involve pot, drugs, drinking, and sex. Within this search for approval, they look for like-minded individuals and the issues begin to expand.

As a Caregiver and paraeducator, I could sense their loss of independence, freedom, and choice and it became my job to begin a process of undoing what was done, which entails a level of trust and preparedness to be tested in ways unimaginable.

What I found was that the simple task of giving them choices and respecting these choices was vital. Their knowledge of the consequences of their choices, good or bad, and knowing what they were, plus being consistent was vital. They had to be ready to take ownership of the choices they made. That may sound easy, but in many cases it takes years to get to a relatively comfortable point with them. They are with me only a few hours a day, and at the end of that time they go back to the place where their independence was limited whether it be a class or home.

Another avenue I use to break through the ice is finding out what their passion is. It can be a lifesaver in many situations. It is hard to get them to tell you their true passion, as they think girls or drugs are their real passions sometimes. When they do divulge their true passion, meaning something that sparks them and grabs their interest, their outlook on school and life in general changes to one that is positive. One of my kids loved race cars and talked about them a lot. One day he felt like he was losing his independence in the class and felt cornered. I took him outside, and we looked at all the cars in the parking lot. I asked him which one he thought was the hottest, and which would be good to convert into a race car. He felt like the chains had been cut and he could think freely. Little things like that can make a difference.

What I found was after a while of working with them, they could not wait to come work with me and learn new things. I had to be consistent with the three A's: accessible, approachable and available. When I saw them in the community, they would seek me out, and I always got a hug. Many of my former students have helped me in caregiving situations and offered to help me restore the 16-room Victorian home I have purchased to hopefully turn it into a place for respite for TBI (Traumatic Brain Injury).

So, in the end, I feel there is hope. Many people say that kids today will never amount to anything but I have witnessed the opposite. One of the key components to success with kids and especially teens is to instill a sense of ownership and independence in them, something we all cherish as individuals and as a nation.

Independence is learned, earned and yearned for in our society. If we take the time to first ask if they need help and then act appropriately, this will be the beginning of our success

LEGACY

According to the Webster dictionary, legacy is "money or property that is left to relatives, friends or associates after one dies or leaves". It also has a deeper meaning. While someone is alive, it has to do with the things they accomplish, do for a living, encouraging others to do better, how they relate to others. It can include, Leaving a box of letters to people you love after you die, books and other things that depict who you are or were, writing a book as I am doing, songwriters, singers and musicians who leave music you cannot get out of your head. It can also relate to memories in your life, how you teach, whether you are a teacher or not, work and associate with our human neighbors, relatives and cultures. Items, encounters and events that you will leave behind for someone else to use, read, learn from or encapsulate into their personality are just some of the tools that can be used. One thing that is vital to the longevity of our legacy is how we are with our youth as a mentor, teacher, guide and friend.

In the realm of caregiving, sickness, and incapacity, and suddenly you are in a situation of panic and fear that you may not have long on this earth, it is easy to see how we might have the need to complete as much as possible and get one's life in order. We also may be concerned about how we will be remembered. No one wants to be remembered for dying from complications of HIV when they have had such an amazing life. Some may have had not so great a life and no time to atone for their mistakes. Sometimes, the legacy we wish to live and leave when we die can be rudely interrupted and shattered by one single word, incident, or action. In the case of people who have been upstanding citizens for most or all of their lives, and something happens where they make a choice that will alter their legacy forever and be the one thing people remember them for, we have to realize that it is a choice. Society, no matter how God-like or good like they are, will remember the one thing they did wrong and hold on to that. "I never thought he would have done that. He was such a good soul; I don't know what happened. I cannot and will not believe he did this." These are some of the things people say about people they respect. Many were blindsided by what they did or said that went against the social norms of decency or they may have harmed someone. Legacy is unpredictable yet with an element of controllability.

Many of the people I worked with during the HIV/AIDS crisis and individuals who were battling cancer introduced me to this fear of leaving their kids and not leaving a legacy of love or strength that they wished they could have. "No time left to change," was a common phrase during our conversations. Even for Mark and so many others at that time, the fear was that because AIDS was such a stigmatized part of the social fabric that they would only be remembered as someone who had AIDS. When someone dies of complications due to AIDS or drugs or cancer or diabetes, we say what they died of when reference to them. It seems to define who they were. Not fair, is it?

This bothered me and led me to think about my legacy. For many of us, we do not talk about our history, personal feelings, and accomplishments unless we are writing a resume or trying to impress others. As a father and grandfather, I would like to believe that what I do with my family and what I express to them will make a difference for the better in their lives. Just recently I watched the "March For Our Lives" in Washington and around the world. What I saw was the culmination of the legacy left to these kids from their parents and parenting, their listening to the stories of their grandparents, the effect on them of the legacy of the social media used in a productive way, and the effect the teachers all over the world. These teachers who are underpaid for producing the quality of students who have emerged from their efforts. This is the next generation of leaders and we are partly responsible for how they turn out in the end. In the 60s and 70s, it was the youth who changed our thinking and society fought back, calling them hippies and druggies. Now we joke about that time with phrases like, "I don't remember the 60s". The legacy that happened with the movement for racial equality and the Vietnam protests made a difference, even if at times it does not seem like it. What we do with that legacy and how we progress is vital. The legacy they left us was to be conscious enough about social injustice and corruption, to be able to think before we act. Now 50 years later we are seeing a resurgence of this phenomenon that I am sure will not go away soon. The movement Black Lives Matter, fight against school shootings and the response to police shootings has reopened the plea that was so loud in the 60s to a fever pitch as we, a society so diverse and yet divided, take what was accomplished then for granted. A lot of what is happening now is being made visible by the youth, blacks, and women, as it was in the 60s, not the adults who are too busy trying to keep the status quo. The youth have the freshness and clarity of mind, and are not tainted by many years of mistakes, experiences and just living. Have you ever heard the phrase, "I was so into making a difference and then life happened?" When one has a job, time is a factor, as is commitment. Of course, as in the sixties, we hear the oppositions to protests, "Get a job!" "Go home to mommy!" "Go back to class!" or "Get a life!" These young people see things in an unobstructed view and act on it. We sometimes forget that they are our future and if they are making this much of a difference now, what can they do later? But remember that there is always a fork in the road, and it can go both ways. Open your history books. It is all there.

Having the opportunity to talk to so many who were living with an illness that could kill them, opened my eyes to new possibilities. I spent many hours listening to people whose legacies were amazing, and learned how they had the control to create the legacy they wanted to leave. Many said, "And then life happened," but they were able to conquer the restrictions of life and move on. When one becomes ill, we panic. How sick will I get? How bad will it get? If it is a terminal illness, how long will I have? The tears and fears that accompany all this will be a roller coaster ride of emotion. How will it affect my family? These questions will pop in and out of your life until it becomes part of that phrase, life just happened, I just got sick, I never thought I would get

Cancer, Leukemia, Alzheimer's, Dementia, Diabetes or an accident. It just happened. At this point, most of them were so blinded by the present situation that they did not see their legacies and were mostly afraid that this illness or event would be the only thing they would be remembered for. Now the trick is to overcome change that and move to a higher level of consciousness and control. It's not an easy task, and it also depends on your support system. One of the biggest fears of people whose illness is terminal or irreversible is that they will have to battle it alone. Having a strong support system who will have the patience and the willingness to listen to who you are and what your needs are right now so that you can be in control of what you want to leave as your legacy, can make all the difference in the world.

You can be specific as to what your legacy will be, and who you want it to affect. This is the start of focusing your attention on the legacy process, which can have an amazing effect on the quality of your life. Using this to your advantage can be a life-altering event for most of us. Clarity is one of the benefits indeed. I have been conscious of this process for many years, and everything I do and the people I associate with or do not associate with has made a big difference in the individual legacies I leave. With each student, associate, and group I encounter, I make an effort to look at the legacy I am leaving. I am not perfect, and if you ask some people I have not had good relationships I am sure I will be referred to as an ASS. In these cases, I look at how much energy would be expended in rectifying the situation versus just letting it go. The key is that I must make an initial effort to rectify it. Unfortunately, there are two or more sides to this, and some things will not change.

To get back to the Legacy Program, as the peer education coordinator for several HIV/AIDS groups in the 90s, my job was to teach each group of people who were HIV positive how to comfortably talk about the issues connected to their illness, stigma, social acceptance and the fears of the illness in the community. I was extremely concerned that their fear of not being able to make a difference in the lives of the people they wanted to leave a legacy for would be a barrier to their success in talking to the community. So that was my first order of business, to explore the legacy they wanted to leave and to whom. This would take weeks and sometimes months to process, as each person was different. I had throughout three years about forty people who I worked with in the Legacy Program. There were many more who signed up, but they were still in the "too much life getting in the way" part of the experience, so their attendance was limited.

As each person went through the process, they would present questions at every level. Many of the questions were based on the, "what it can do for me". As each question was asked, I would take that question and create an individualized process for each person. Some wanted their children to know who they were and how much they loved them, as the children were quite young and were not totally aware of the issues and their depths. There are so many things that can be created for something like this - writing, poems, letters, video and material creations like paintings and sculptures that can be left for them. I have incorporated many different avenues to attain success in this area. Many of the people I worked with have come up with their own ways to leave their legacy. The program became a joint venture and very individualized. The questions were basic and the answers were deep and troubling at times, but when all is said and done, those who took it seriously, thanked me for allowing them a to peek at the possibilities that were out there to make a difference.

Since my days in NYC and Yonkers, I have found that most of the people who wanted to know more about the program were people with children. Many did not see them often, like people who lived a long way from their families, older people, military personnel, people who own companies and travel, and parents who are separated and have lost control of their influence in their child's life. I began to share this program, or at least the contents of it, with people I have encountered along the way. One by one, I saw positive feedback with great results and thanks for sharing it. In this chapter, I will allow you a peek at the guts of it, and it will be up to you to adapt it to your situation. It can be adapted to anyone's world, so I am confident that it can work for anyone who tests its validity. I have also been exploring the possibilities with the criminal justice system, as many of the inmates are in a place where they think they have no control as the bars and walls are the barriers to their success with their children and life in general. It also has possibilities with the behavior and situations the inmates will experience as human beings which could be an asset to restorative justice.

So, take some time to study the following paragraphs and see if you can apply it to where you are in life and what you would like to leave as a legacy.

Legacy

What is Legacy?

- Legacy is a program that originally was focused on people who were "dying" or "living," if you will, from/with complications from HIV.
- It eventually expanded to people who were dying from cancer, diabetes, Alzheimer's, and any illness that is considered terminal.
- To successfully use this program, one must change the word "dying from" to "living with."
- It is a program designed to allow a person to look at who they are, or where and how they are received in the community and family. Knowing this, they can take control of the legacy they would like to leave for those whom they will leave behind.
- Later I realized that it can be adapted to many other situations like how people see others, organizations, companies and even government. Many have taken this program and used it to help leave a legacy for their children they cannot see at present from divorce, illness, military, work, or just living apart for any reason.
- Legacy is the quality of life, structure, and product that will be left to someone else or to the community after someone leaves, is transferred out of an institution, or dies.

Does everyone leave a legacy? Yes.
Can we leave one while we are alive? Yes.
Is it complete? No.
Can a legacy continue to grow after one dies? Yes
Are all legacies good? No.

Examples are everywhere. Just look around at the historical statues in Washington and all the capitals in the US. Small towns are full of people who have done incredible things in their lives and who have changed the faces of towns, cities, and the country. Yet there is a dark side to legacy. You can see the intentional slaughter of humans and the destruction of the infrastructure of whole countries. WWI and WWII, Vietnam, and the legacy of slavery in many countries and the US, are striking examples of how terrifying a legacy can be. These are bad or negative legacies that have, in most cases, happened because of greed, profit and the idea that some people are superior while others are expendable. They become the enemy, and human nature has dictated for centuries that we must conquer or suppress our enemies. This idea has gone back as far as the dawn of humans. It is a natural phenomenon branded in the building of many cultures and in the name of survival of the fittest, and many times we call this progress. In most of these instances, it was the purposeful plot and execution of a process to attain land and greatness, or just to eliminate or use a population that is different from whoever is in power. We see it in today's society daily.

On the upside of legacy, we also can purposefully create a legacy of peace, love, and goodness that can transcend time and greatness. Look at the poets who have inspired us to do great and loving things. Songs help us become inspired and to move on to a peaceful solution. Books that are road maps to the good life and good healthy living, and even love letters we send to family and friends and loved ones inspire us to move on after a tragedy or death.

Of course, we can look at the legacies of some people, like those great icons of our cultures who within the dark entanglement of their lives have been overlooked. Because slavery had become part of the culture and was accepted as necessary, we now look at that era with fresh and disceiminating eyes. Here in the US recently, we have begun to dismantle the statues and symbols of our past. I am sure if we look deep enough into the past and the lives of the people today who have amazing legacies, we will find flaws. We are human. Humans are not perfect, and we must understand that with all the good that someone does or quotes that inspire us to be the best we can be, we will find blemishes. It is up to us to gather as much of the good that can raise us up and cherish these gems of wisdom, and put aside (but not forget) the blemishes that come along with them. The idea is to inspire ourselves and to recreate ourselves from the goodness that was left to us by our past as well as our present, and learn lessons from the errors of the past.

So, when someone is affected by an illness or another situation that has opened up the possibility of leaving behind memories for our children, friends, and citizens that do not reflect our truth, we can begin the amazing journey of legacy. This journey is not easy; it is time-consuming and it is frustrating, as people who are going through the twelve-step program can attest to, yet it is still amazing and wonderful when the goals have been attained and a legacy is created. These goals are created by the one who is attempting to leave a legacy. One of the biggest hurdles to climb over is looking at ourselves and who we are. All through this journey, you will find questions and some amazing and eye-opening answers. Some of us will be disappointed at times, and all I can say is that if you truly want to create the legacy you wish to leave, you must move on and conquer those hurdles. Put them behind you, but remember they exist. To not acknowledge them would be dangerous, as it would render an incomplete or false legacy that others will have to tangle with or could recognize in some cases. That would be a tarnish that would be difficult to erase.

We live in a wonderfully rich time to create a legacy. The computer and all the technology we have can be an amazing tool for this journey, as you will see. Yet just the ability to handwrite a letter to your children or friends who may receive it before or after your death, can be one of the most welcome pieces of the legacy you are about to leave. Since I have become aware of this journey in the last 20 years, I became conscious of my legacy, and every person I meet I try to purposefully do things, say things, and leave the best legacy I can. I am not perfect, and there are those I have met who I have left a less than perfect legacy because of their refusal or incapacity to accept me, or the legacy I wish to leave. Their constant judging or searching for something bad I have done or potentially could do is a big pothole in the road. We all have a choice to deal with it or put it aside. Everything in legacy is a choice.

Many have said to me that my belief in legacy is selfish, self-centered, narcissistic, and only serves the purpose of making me feel good about myself. Granted, it does feel good and does build my self-esteem up to a nice level but why is that not okay, unless done in excess? I also look at how it has changed the people around me and changed what they might aspire to.

I did not say it was an easy process. It will bring to light situations and people who will want to put a wrench in your process. One such time put me in a depression with a depth I have never experienced. I was working for a non-profit, which was the best job I have ever had. It had all the components of my existence and experiences, all in one job. Education, retail, helping the poor, the arts, connecting with many agencies who have the same goals of helping others, and management were embedded in this job I was lucky enough to have. In the end, I was told that there was a budget crunch and my job was eliminated, but before they let me go they praised me for all the good I had done and for my accomplishments, which made the fall of being let go a lot harder. I went into such a period of questioning myself on unemployment, which I had never done in my 70 years, and depression I had no prior experience with. I also found out from the horse's mouth that there were several people who wanted me out and made my job a miserable experience in the last few weeks of my stay there. The legacy I was trying to leave with that company was suddenly out of my control, but to this day people remember my stay there and the fun we had making the place work.

During this time I had to evaluate who I was, what I had done, and how I would handle everything, plus take a fresh look at the legacy journey I was on. This was a true test for me, as I always had at least two jobs, plus a lot of nonprofits I worked with over the years. I began to watch TV during one of the most depressing springs and all the political upheaval, the scandals, and sad events began to encapsulate my mind and thinking. I became a recluse, and it was not until my friend Alex Anastasi-Hill, who worked in the nonprofit I was let go from, got me to go out for some beers and give me a pep talk that I began the task of getting back on my feet. One of the problems of job hunting was that I was 69, and even though I had all the experience in the world, everyone was looking for some young kid they could mold, develop and would not die of old age in a few years. I had just experienced ageism or age discrimination. It had to happen eventually. I thought of getting mad, but once I began to accept that there is that part of society still in existence and there was little I could do about it, I was fine. I also met a young man, Bogdan Kulbida from the Ukraine, who was a neighbor and has become one of the best friends one could meet. He was bright, young, and had a passion to succeed I have seldom seen. His goal was to open his own business. Yet there was a dark place in his heart. He had experienced divorce, and his son was in Ukraine, and the distance was making it hard to talk to him. I told him over a few beers about the legacy program, and that no matter how much he was not physically in his son's life, he could create a legacy for his son that would transcend all his pain at the present time. He now has set up a legacy of daily talks to his son on the computer, recording what he is thinking at the time, how much his son means to him, and why he cannot be there. Amazing. The question came up, "What if he does not accept this when he gets older?" I had to let him know that he had no control of that, and it would be up to his son to accept or not accept all that he is doing. It is still a legacy, and when, at some time in his son's life, he becomes wise and aware of how valuable all this is, he will accept it in his own time and on his terms. There are some tricks I have up my sleeve that could guarantee that he will listen to them.

This is the uncertainty of legacy. You can do all you want, but it is up to who receives the information to utilize it and appreciate it.

There are three questions presented to you in the legacy program which all take a lot of soul searching and probing within your soul.

Question #1

"If you were to leave my presence, leave this room, or leave this life, how do you think you will be remembered by me, people you know, and the world?"

This is a question that will need some interaction between you and the people you know. I usually suggest, (and in the course I allow), several weeks of intense investigating and questioning and note-taking. Most people are uncomfortable doing a lot of this, and it is up to you to follow through to succeed. It is designed to get a glimpse of what people see in you, how they react to you, and why they feel that way. I always suggest to the person asking these questions that they go into this with an understanding that they may be disappointed, and to ask those who are being asked to be as truthful as they can comfortably be. Let them know that it is ok if they have negative feelings, as they can become constructive bricks that will build the reality you need to know before going on.

If you feel too uncomfortable about this and you are not ready to hear any negative responses, please do not continue this session. You may assume you know the answers to the first question and move to the next.

During the first session, we do a brainstorming of things that can be done to make the process easier. We practice on each other in the class, but as an individual you may be on your own unless you find someone who you can trust to practice with. This can last 2 to 3 weeks or more if needed. The key is to take what you hear at face value and do not judge yourself harshly. The answers you may hear are only one person's perspective that you may not have seen in yourself. I asked a person whom I had met a while back, and something he said caused me to examine my actions. He said, "You say you are going to do something and either you forget and never do it, or you remember too late. You do it a lot." I tried to connect it to the mini-stroke I had, but I still needed to look at it. Again, if you think it will cause stress in your relationships, please do a self-examination of who you are and move to the next question.

Once you have done this first step and you are comfortable with what your findings are and that people have been truthful with you, you are ready for the next question.

Question #2

"If you leave my presence, leave this room, or leave this life, how would you like to be remembered?"

This question takes a lot longer to study. To look at the life you presently lead is important to explore with the people you associate with. Take note of your ups and downs in all aspects of your life, your passions, your dislikes and likes. Study your belief systems in all areas of your life, how you feel about other belief systems, what your strengths are and especially check out your weaknesses as many times that is what shows up the most to others. Noticing how you present yourself to others, your health, your dress style, such as, do you always wear jeans or well-cut pants and shirts, hairstyle, and all the things that others will see first can give you a physical picture you can work with. Would you like to be remembered as a kind and generous person, cold and precise, or a person who will listen rather than talk? These are many of the things I had to look at and had to change to get to where I wanted to be. It is not an easy process and may take many weeks to do it. The key for me was to take one evening and make the first list that came to my mind. I put it aside and did some thinking. When I felt like continuing, I took the list out and added to it, or made an outline of the list and what it would entail. For me, outlines were the easiest to work with. One thing that helped me in the personal presentation area was to listen to people and what they said when I wore certain things. I found when I wore white shirts or sweaters, people commented that I looked great. Khaki pants instead of jeans was another story. It was not until I had worn white and khaki so much that some questioned if I had any other clothes that I realized I was overdoing it.

I spent a month doing the preliminary work and was very critical of everything I listed. I then had a very close friend who knew what I was doing help me go through it and tell me how realistic it was. Having fresh eyes was important to me at that time. Then, I picked out people I wanted to leave legacies to and tweaked what needed tweaking on an individual basis.

In many ways it was self-centered, but it was only foolish to those who did not think that leaving a legacy was important or just did not care what others thought, which is fine. There are times when I could not care less what others think, but most of the time I believe legacy to be important, amazing, and vital to those we love.

I realized that it was helping me become a better person. Yet, I was told it was not the real me. When I looked at the real me that took so many years to create, which is the one they saw, it was done in the same way but unconsciously. While constructing the recreated me, I kept the basic beliefs and my soul for the most part, but dressed it up and began to look at how I wanted to make a difference, and how all these things on the list were a way to get that done. For the past 25 years, I have dressed well (except in the morning when there is only me to scare), tried to organize most of my life, and tried to deal with all the little things that hold me back from the legacy I want to leave. The organizational part of my life, I am still working on. ADD does not help the situation either.

I am sure most would consider me a hoarder of antiques, and I still have excuses for each item. But that is a bigger story, and one that will be part of the 16 room Victorian that was mentioned earlier. I want to recreate this house to be a place of respite for people with TBI and be part of the solution and not the problem. Some of my former students have had accidents from skiing, hiking or car crashes. They all have Traumatic Brain Injuries. I try to meet with them once a month for pizza and make sure their services are in place, and they are doing ok. They were the ones who suggested I buy a place where they could stay for respite instead of a hospital or nursing home where they lose their independence. Again, this is all part of the legacy I wish to leave.

Now when I leave a meeting, I make sure I am heard and remembered in a good way. I also make sure I have listened to everyone without judgement. For people who are Caregivers, it becomes a bit more intense. Keeping a smile on, listening to their needs, and making sure that you do not say things that may hurt or embarrass those being taken care of. For those who are ill it is even harder, and that is why I try to include the Caregiver and family in the explanation and process of this program. Most people cannot see how important it is to make sure they leave a legacy and to who, especially if they are ill or losing ground with the effects of Dementia and Alzheimer's. That is why it is so important to be sensitive to the needs of the ones being cared for who are looking to leave a legacy.

Once you have found all the things you want to create in your life to make that legacy a truth, you can let it sit. I suggest a specific file on the computer with all the lists and results. I also suggest going back and reading what you have several times. For those who like pen and paper, keep it all in one notebook. Give yourself a pat on the back for getting this far and relax. You should be proud of yourself.

Question #3

"Now that you know the answers to both previous questions, what is it that you need to do on a daily, weekly, monthly, or yearly basis to make the legacy you are looking to leave become real?"

This is a tough one. There is an infinite list of things that could be done or discussed at this point. It mainly depends on what your talents are, what your passion is, and who you wish to leave a legacy to. For me, it is now primarily this book, but for years it was dealing with how I was perceived as a Caregiver in so many situations. I had to look at my strong points and especially my weak points. What was I doing that I could do better? What was I doing that I need to delete? What was I not doing that I should do? It was a tough one indeed, as I had to admit I was not up to par in some areas and needed to take a good look at them. I can be stubborn with myself a lot and do not like to be wrong, but I have always taken responsibility for the things I did wrong. I had to look at all the guidelines of caregiving, legally and morally. It was a lot of soul searching. Many of the "ah-ha" moments that occurred during this journey were the teaching moments that would throw me into the next section.

There are so many ways to leave a legacy such as in the situation my friend Bogdan was in the US from the Ukraine. His son is still in the Ukraine and he felt that just calling him once in a while or sending him presents was not enough. He is a programmer and has worked with computers for some time. He opened a company in Seattle, Washington, and his company name has his son's name in it, as one way to start the legacy. He has such an opportunity to use the technological tools at his fingertips.

Creating an online diary of his thoughts, ideas, passions, dreams, and feelings for his son who is now five, was one of his most powerful tools. Even if something happens to Bogdan, he has already left something. When his son gets to an age to make decisions, he can see his diary. If Bogdan creates a video diary, he will see his father talking to him directly. Anyone in this situation can leave one of these written or recorded, and leave years of conversation to those who cannot yet understand. One of the most effective methods was to record the conversations of he and his son talking to each other. His son will be able to hear what he sounded like at 5, 6, and so on. What I would give to hear conversations with my Dad and me at that age.

I had always envied the children of film stars who can watch their parents as they were when they were younger. I doubt that they understood what a legacy they were leaving their children, as it was just a job they did.

Here is a list of tools you can use, things you can create and things to do for your legacy:

- The computer, iPad or phone to record yourself daily, write, or take video of who you are.

- The old fashioned pen. Leaving a legacy in your own handwriting does make it more personal.
- The camera. As a photographer, I was able to record my son Homer's life. That act alone made such a difference in our relationship even though we were apart for many years, but I always took my camera with me when I was with him. Now it is so much cheaper to do with digital, and it can all be stored on the computer or other devices. Look at the legacy Ansel Adams left with his photos of nature and landscape shots that are now there for all time. He was one of my mentors.
- Cars. I have a friend who worked on rebuilding cars for members of his family.
- Art. Leaving artwork that you have created. I have some paintings a friend did for me, and he would have (and many times did) put them in the trash. I saved them, and they are now precious pieces of the friendship I had with him. In cases when the person became famous, the value of finding lost Picassos or sketches from the hand of one of the great writers or painters is so important and a great way to see how they developed their ideas. Father Burt spent many months reading scripture to a boy with Down Syndrome who lived in an institution. Each time he came back, Andre had a piece of artwork for him. I have a collection from that experience and pictures of him and Burt chatting. Eventually he stopped drawing and no one knew why. But for that short period, a legacy was left.
- Music. Writing a song or piece of music for someone can be an amazing legacy. How many times do you have the experience of music that relates to an experiences in your life?
- Poetry, which is one of the things I do, is a direct link in the creative sense to the person it is about. This can also be accomplished with a short story.
- Writing letters and putting them away, in the cases where people are at odds with each other, can after death or a tragedy be such a healer, and the legacy it will leave is priceless.
- Presentation, as in learning how to present yourself in the manner and dress you wish people to remember you by. If

you are the "bad boy or girl" and you want that to be part of your legacy, it can be done. On the other side, keeping yourself neatly dressed, hair combed and presentable in that fashion, will leave a legacy of self-esteem and poise. Think of who you are and how you want to present that. Willard Scott was the first Ronald McDonald and was Claribel in the Howdy Doody years. So, you can go as far as you want with this.

- Gardening. My dad and Burt's dad were both gardeners. They left us such a wealth of knowledge and the legacy they left was the gardens they created and how people remember their wonderful flowers. My dad was a member of the Gladioli Society, and I remember him dragging us to all the meetings and events and giving us some of the most powerful first-hand knowledge of this species. It became one of my first 4-H projects, and I did several demonstrations on it. When I went to Brazil, I passed on a lot of that knowledge, as I was in an agriculturally-based program. They were impressed, and now in some circles, I am remembered as the flower guy down there.

- Teachers have one of the most amazing and profound platforms for legacy. Who doesn't remember the one you disliked the most? Legacy can go both ways and, in most cases, teachers are not aware of the process of legacy. Can you imagine if they did how amazing they would be? We also remember the teachers who made the most difference in our lives.

- In the ministry and priesthood, there is a special place for legacy. Fr. Burt, "The Heart of Yonkers," was and is remembered as the storyteller. His philosophy was that you can preach a sermon and you will either bore them to death, or they will never remember it, but if you tell a story, they will remember the story better than the sermon. Also, how many Catholics can remember the kindness of the nuns, or the Nun Nazi as I had called one who would yell and beat her stick on her hand if we talked or were out of line? Damn. We were only ten years old.

- Profession. In olden days if you fixed clocks, you were the clockmaker, and there was the baker, silversmith, toymaker, candlestick maker, knight of the round table, and all the professions right up to the King. That was the legacy you were given, and it outlived you. Does King Arthur ring a bell?

I am sure you can come up with many other tools and arenas where legacy can be effective. Take some time and look at these facilities and see how you can use them. Personalize them and make them yours.

There are many sides and opinions to this process and legacy itself. I was listening to a radio talk show and one of the guests said, why would anyone spend so much on legacy. If you look at the sports and entertainment world, the only people who care about the legacy they leave and have a vested interest in who they are would be the people, stars or sports figure themselves. This is their job and much of the legacy they leave has already happened. Yet they also had to work hard on it. I am not saying that they all have not put their all into it, but in some cases they were at the right place at the right time. That field goal, the book that came out at the right time or the song they sang may have become an anthem for someone else. John Lennon with giving Peace A Chance, or Peter, Paul, and Mary during the 60s all with their protest songs along with Bob Dylan, Bobby Darin, Tom Paxton, and Pete Seeger. If you listen today, you may still hear them whispering, or "blowing in the wind of change". These are great legacies that just happened with a lot of preparation but it was not on purpose. Some were lucky, and some knew they were involved in something bigger than all of us. What is this new generation of young people going to leave as a legacy? What is your legacy?

Legacy has a wide range of directions as to where it can go and how to get there. It is a very individual and personal experience and can take you far or nowhere at all, depending on how much you want to invest. The people we remember in history, literature, science, art, and mathematics, not to mention all the social giants that left such amazing legacies, invested a lifetime of invention, purpose, and stamina in attaining the legacy. I do not expect this is for everyone, but anyone can do it. I especially like to see parents and relatives taking the opportunity to leave a video legacy at least, as it would be such an amazing "ah ha" moment for their children to see and hear them, and to hear themselves if you record them too. Think about someone you miss who is gone and what you would give to see you and them interacting. Many times, people forget the voices of loved ones and how they looked and acted. This would be one amazing gift.

DIGNITY VS. CARING TOO MUCH

From the time in my life when I protected my neighbor with Down Syndrome, (we were both about 10 years old), to the present, I have always felt the need we all have for a little dignity in our lives. Sometimes I would see Charles get bullied where the kids would surround him and push him around. He would think they were playing a game and laugh. Several times I had to jump in and told him to run and I got the bullying. It was one of my first attempts to give someone back a little of their dignity.

What is dignity? Dignity can be as simple as allowing a person the dignity of making decisions.

It can be respecting someone's wishes, or just doing something to make a situation more pleasant or respectable. In many cases for me, it has been allowing my charge to do as much for themselves as possible and not trying to do too much for them. I had a student who used a leg brace. When I had to transport him, he would wait for me to open the door as he had injured his arm also. One day I asked him to open the door, because my arms were full. I purposely did that to see if he would open the door. He opened it with little effort. From then on, he opened his own doors and pulled himself up on the car seat. Later he told me that he was glad that I did that, because it gave him a sense of ownership of who he was and what he did. His reliance was wearing on others, and he could see it.

One thing I used to do with Mark, Frank, Elsie, and Burt was make sure their hair was combed, they were shaved, and cleaned when visitors came to see them. No one wants to be visited by someone when they are having a bad hair day.

When you show respect, it can be allowing them to talk for themselves. I found many times I would take Burt and Mark to the hospital and when questions were asked by the doctor, I found myself answering for them, which in turn frustrated them and the doctor. There were times when the doctor told me sternly, "I asked 'him', not you." I found myself being overprotective, which can be stifling to them and leads them to feel helpless with whatever is going on. They feel they have no say and it only compounds the pain. I am not saying that when they ask for help to tell them to help themselves, although there were times I thought about it, but I would always suggest to them to see if they can do it themselves or figure out a way to do it, and then help them if they couldn't. I know the feeling of being helpless, as having had a mini-stroke debilitated me for a while.

As a Caregiver, it is easy to jump in and take control, and at times can seem a bit rude to the person being cared for. You want everything to work out right for them. I have seen it in hospitals when the nurse may be stern about something and it may sound like the patient is being scolded. When Burt was in the hospital, I noticed several times when he was losing control of some bodily functions and sometimes did not know it had happened. The nurse came in and innocently said, "Oh no, not again." Burt felt like he had done something wrong, and then had to be tossed around in the bed to correct the situation. (For me it was a glimpse into the future as I was his Caregiver and I did not want to be Nurse Ratchet from the 1975 film "One Flew Over the Cuckoo's Nest")

After talking to the head nurse on that floor, she apologized and said that sometimes we say what we feel and do not realize who is listening. This is dangerous for the patient, client, or person being cared for, as it can disclose information that could jeopardize their welfare. When I worked for The Sharing Community in Yonkers, I found out that by just having a picture of someone in my office anyone can misinterpret that, thinking the person in the picture was HIV positive. It happened once when I had a group pic of some students who helped volunteer for us and myself. A community member who was about to help us with a project noticed someone in the picture and decided not to hire him after seeing him in the pic. I heard about the situation and called him up and told him that the boy was only a volunteer. I then proceeded to take all the pictures out of my office. As a photographer for camps to help people with disabilities, cancer, and AIDS, I had to be careful and take photos of only those who had signed a release and only used them in the slide show presentation that was put to music at the end of camp. This applies to agencies who work with mental health (which is where I work now), and even schools where Special Ed is a program.

So, be conscious of who you are with. Know the person well before letting anyone know who you work with, if you say anything at all. When in a one on one situation or with other coworkers and a client, be careful of your words. People are sensitive to many things, and to keep their dignity intact you need to be aware and knowledgeable about interpersonal relationships. Be careful of over-caring or intruding on their rights.

I have also been in situations where workers, camp counselors, teachers, and hospital personnel sit together and chit chat amongst themselves. Many times, they will be whispering and may inadvertently look at someone. Now the person they glanced at may think they are being discussed in the whispers. This can cause clients and co-workers undue stress. It is not an easy job in many respects when working in groups like this. When I was a manager at a retail establishment, one of the first things I noticed was that it was easy to disrespect others unknowingly just because this is normal in their private life. My first job was to warn every one of the workers and volunteers that if I see someone or hear of anyone disrespecting a customer, volunteer, or worker, I will give them a warning. I gave out many warnings in the beginning, but had to be patient as this is not an easy task, knowing what the community was like. Eventually, dignity was restored, and customers came back and enjoyed the environment.

The dictionary says dignity is also, "bearing, conduct, or speech indicative of self-respect or appreciation of the formality or gravity of an occasion or situation." Treating clients, as people who are sensitive and have feelings should be a no-brainer. Yet we are all different and are brought up differently, similar to the difference in cultures. In some cultures, it is polite to burp after eating or slurp your soup from a bowl. It is a constant battle. Everyone I know at work has caught themselves in a violation, even of the smallest magnitude. It is not a norm in society, as we live in a world where survival of the fittest can sometimes take precedence and beating your opponent is what matters most. Having to switch gears all the time makes it difficult.

WE'VE COME A LONG WAY, BABY

Being protective can be a good thing, especially when safety and injury can be a major issue. With the elderly, it is a touchy subject. From my own experience, I had fallen, tripping over the dog. I hit a porcelain umbrella stand and broke my nose. Luckily, my son Homer was visiting from New York. I got up off the floor. All I could see was the blood, and I noticed my nose was off to the side. I quickly put it back in place and told my son to take me to the hospital. While I was there, I was questioned about how safe it was for me to go home, as I was reaching 70. For me, it was humiliating, as I am a very independent person and do not like people taking care of me. I was asked again, and my son was asked many times as well. Do I need a call button? Can I climb stairs? Does someone live with me? Having someone live with me would be even worse, as we would probably kill each other. I was losing my dignity brick by brick.

On the other hand, it can become dangerous for the person being cared for. Keeping a positive and progressive relationship and being sensitive to that, as well as not depriving the person of a chance to speak for themselves (or in other words, losing one's self), can be a vital part of the caregiving process and success.

While working with several individuals who had limited vocabulary, I found myself speaking to them again and again until one of them yelled one of the few words he knew: "No!" and later, "Go away!" Another "ah-ha" moment I live to tell about. I eventually had to realize my limits as well as theirs. Yet after 22 years of being the Caregiver of one of them, as well as para educator and friend, I still find myself falling into that pothole of being too protective, which infringes on his dignity and self-esteem. That need for dignity and justice has followed me all my life. While volunteering for a youth group called STAR, which started as a group who took kids with disabilities out bowling, to the movies, picnics, dances and a host of other activities to help them be a part of the community social network, I encountered some situations with myself and others who did not listen or thought they knew better. One of the kids mentioned to me that he hated summers, because his brother could go camping and he could not, and he had to stay home. This got me thinking, and I saw that his dignity and self-esteem were affected. As a group, we were very protective of them. We could only help them with the limited resources we had. Eventually, I would become the founder and first director of Camp Happyness.

Unfortunately, this was the 60s, and there was still the attitude that they would be better off warehoused in an institution, out of sight and out of mind. We were only working with the kids whose families who were strong enough to keep them in the community.

One of the first jobs I had was as an attendant in a cottage at Ladd School, now shut down, which was a warehouse for people whom society felt were repulsive, odd, too high maintenance, and were commonly referred to as "Retarded." That was a blanket label for so many disabilities. One of my early attempts to restore dignity was at this school or institution. I also became very protective of the residents of the cottage. Some of them were quite smart, but having been in this environment for so long, their social interactions and daily habits were evidence of prolonged seclusion. I would challenge them all the time mentally and physically, and show them as much love and understanding as I could muster under the circumstances. Many of my coworkers, who had been there some time, kept reminding me I was wasting my time. They would tell me not to become too close to them, as their future is questionable and will be here the rest of their lives. I still remember her face and that statement. When people used to call these institutions funny farms, it was because it was like a farm and the livestock were human. Man, we have come a long way. I have to keep reminding myself that when I work with mental health and get discouraged about the slow progress in getting things done, or when funding is dropped and the clients end up suffering, that we are so much more advanced than we were then. We have come a long way, baby.

The cottage I was in had an inside day room where the floor and walls were tiled, and the floor had two drains in it. Doors and windows were always locked, and the smell of urine was prevalent. Anyone who has worked in one of these relics of the past will know what I mean. I hate to say it, but it was almost like they were marking their territory. Every evening the room was washed down and disinfected. That is why the room had drains. There was also the occasional spreading of feces, so the disinfectant was a must.

One big problem was that there usually was an 8 to 1 resident/worker ratio. They knew when we were not looking their way, so you had to watch yourself. I asked one of the supervisors "why they are locked up so much". She said, "to protect them from themselves." There were no planned activities, and they were usually spinning on the merry-go-round (or vomit goes round), rocking back and forth, or just sitting staring into space. Many of them had some alertness to what was going on, and I always felt they were planning their escape.

Outside the building was a yard that was enclosed with high fences and less items than were in the day-room. We rarely went out there unless it was a really warm sunny day. I felt sad that they were so enclosed. Most of the time they were only allowed to use the fenced-in area for an hour at a time.

I started to play football or catch with some of the residents who were more verbal than the others. They seemed to know more about what was going on. Granted it was only a few, but I could see them thinking. One day I got them out in the yard, and there was still some snow, so I engaged them in a snowman contest. I have to say, the results were very interesting. What I saw were different personalities out there working together in groups to make something. I hated that they had to be locked up.

Football was a major game for them, and their rules were different from what the NFL had. For instance, if you got the ball you could run anywhere you wanted as long as you did not hit or run anyone over. Over some time the rules got more complicated, and the idea of teams were established, but changing teams in mid-play was an option as long as no one got mad. Little by little, we honed the rules to become more understandable, and they accepted them. I always had in the back of my mind that we would go out in the field next to the cottage where there was grass and no asphalt. Bumps and bruises were common, as well as the effects of gravity.

One day I decided to ask the administration if I could take some of the boys on the grassy field. They seemed interested, but after four weeks of waiting for an answer, I felt it was landing on deaf ears. After the sixth week, I decided to do something on my own. It was time. The boys were ready, and they trusted me.

I came in that day with a few helmets and some knee pads to help with the bumps. I told them that we were going out on the grass and were going to play some ball. They seemed excited, so I got them ready. I told them the rules, and that they had to stay in the lines, I had drawn with rope. Otherwise, we would have to come back in. They all agreed, and we were off.

We assembled at the door to the yard. I let them and all seemed well. We got to the gate, and I could see some of them walking in circles mumbling something, but I assumed they were excited. I knew I did not have any runner history with any of them so I felt confident that they would be okay. I opened the gate slowly, and some of them walked out onto the grass, but some of them just stood with their backs to the fence. This was something new to them. They were not marching to the gym or assembly hall holding hands. They were standing out on the grass by themselves.

I told them to huddle and most did, except for one or two. They were still hugging the fence. I told them that we were going to play ball just like inside the fence, only this time on the grass. After the huddle a couple of them started rolling on the grass, so I did it too, and the others followed. I figured it would make them feel safe. We began to play ball, and within a few minutes, all were participating. We had a good ten-minute game, and we all shook hands and went back in. Apparently, no one noticed us, as we were behind the cottage opposite the admin building.

We attempted this several times with great success, and I was so proud of them. I still had not heard from the administration building, but who cared? It was working, and the house mom loved it. One day we went out and the boys got a little gutsy, and began to throw the ball as hard as they could. The ball went way beyond the cottage and could be seen by the admin offices. When we got back in the cottage, one of the administrators was there to greet us. The boys could not wait to tell him what a great time they had playing football, and invited him to join them next time. As they went in to shower, I was asked to go to the office. There I was greeted with several administrators and an empty chair opposite them.

About ready to poop my pants, I sat down. I was questioned about whether I understood policies and what I was thinking. I explained to them everything that happened, and how I got the trust of the residents. I told him that I thought that we were being too protective of them, and taking away their freedom to choose and explore and learn. These are basic freedoms we all have, and they were only locked up for being different and high maintenance. I said that none of the residents have run away and if they would allow me to do it again, I would invite the administration to join us. I did tell them, however, they had to learn the rules by the seat of their pants.

After the meeting, I was told to return to my work, and they would get back to me. I figured I had at least six weeks to look for a new job, so I did not sweat it. Two days later I was called into the office and met with the same people. They were all in agreement that no harm was done. It was against the rules, and I was to get a three-day suspension for that, but they would like to work with me on getting more "grass time" as they called it, for the residents. I agreed and went on working until I left for Brazil. They even sent four of the residents to Camp Happyness which was a major accomplishment.

What I learned here about being too protective I would carry with me in the back of my mind throughout my life. I would often forget my past lessons but something would spark the memory, and I would back off from being too doding. I assume it is like a mother letting her kids go out on their own. We must let them out of our protective custody and encourage them to be independent and find their way.

We all have that trait, to be protective of something to excess. But if we let go of the rope, it is amazing to see how well they do. When I was taking care of Burt, I was keeping him safe from so many things, and one day one of the store owners in town came by and was asking him questions. Putting on my armor, I answered her. She then said, "I asked Burt. Don't you have anything else to do?" I felt offended and left, but I also remembered that I had to let go.

It was like when I raised pigeons. I did not want to let them out. I heard a famous quote by Kahlil Gibran. "If you love somebody, let them go, for if they return, they were always yours. If they don't, they never were." I freed them and watched them circle the house and watched the rollers tumble to the ground and just missing it, only to fly back up. What a show, and they all came back!

HOMER G AND ME

I have made many references to Homer. Well, this young boy, now a man, has changed my life in so many ways. He has been one of my inspirations to do the legacy program. He has given me so much joy as a son and has shown me that I can be the father I never knew I could have been, and was afraid I could not be.

I met Homer, unknowingly, when I played Santa at The Sharing Community and listened to him tell me what he wanted for Christmas at the age of 8 or 9. I could not have done a good job as I forget what he asked for. His mom frequented the Sharing Community where I worked. A few years later I would meet him at Camp VIVA. My first encounter with him, at the camp was rough as he and another kid were playing soccer and he, purposely or not, kicked my shin and fractured it. (Homer was depicted as Ben in the Camp VIVA section of this book for privacy reasons but Homer gave me permission to use his name here and make the connection.) I had just told him I was going to be his camp counselor for the week. I had a shin brace and a cane to help me cope, which I did not use much. I was also the photographer for the camp and because of that he has now developed an interest in photography. His encounter with Burt and interest in gardening, has led Homer to become an amazing plant man.

I had no plans or interest in having a son, and in fact the thought of being tied down to that responsibility frightened me. I was working closely with his mom, helping her out when I could, and became Homer's guardian ad litem. I had no idea what that would lead to. We became close, and I took him to many basketball games and events

I thought he would like, but more as a big brother than a dad. The relationship we had was special, and I was learning as much from him as he was from me. Burt had a home in Vermont where he would go on weekends, and he would invite Homer to experience the country. I don't think Homer realized how important that experience each month was, and how it would change his life. I even taught him how to drive on the dirt roads of Vermont. Quite an experience, I have to say.

One day I had just come home from a Broadway Show event in NYC and found Homer sitting on the stairs of the rectory. He had his heavy coat on as it was cold, and he didn't look like the spunky Homer I knew. For some reason, his mom was not at home and he had been thrown out of the house. I do not recall the exact incident, but he needed to stay somewhere, so Burt agreed to let him stay in the library of the rectory and told him it was his room till further notice, as it had a convertible couch. The guest room had been turned into my office and was where I did a lot of my projects. So, I was not ready to give that up, especially if I did not know how permanent this would be.

Homer stayed with Burt and me for quite a few years. His mom was not getting any better. She would, in a few years, be in the hospital. Knowing that Homer was about to become a dad, she said to me, "I am not going to die till I get to see the baby." I went down to her room in the hospital and saw a woman who had transformed from a beautiful African American to someone who resembled a holocaust victim. I sat on the edge of her bed for more than an hour, talking about old times and memories we had shared. She suddenly got quiet and said, "Can I ask a favor of you?" I said, "Sure." She said, "Take care of Homer for me, and make sure he grows up to be a good person?" Wow, I was not ready for that. But I told her I would do all I could to make that happen. That was a moment burned in my memory. She got to see her granddaughter and soon after died.

However, long before that, Burt and I had decided we would invite him to live in the Rectory as if he were a son and both of us would share the responsibility. I was mostly living in Vermont and working on Burt's house for his retirement, and Burt was taking the brunt of the responsibility of taking care of Homer in Yonkers. But it was the many trips to Vermont Homer and I took that became special. I had a captive audience and was able to chat with him (or as Homer would say, lecture him) all the way up. Eventually, he would get tired and go in the back of the van and fall asleep on the fold-down seat. For many years he thought it only took an hour or so to get up to Vermont, as he slept through most of it. We had been to Vermont many times but it was not until I let him drive up that he asked me if we were going the right way, as it was taking too long. He became quite aware of how long of a drive it was behind that wheel.

On the way we would stop at the Basketball Hall of Fame in Springfield, Massachusetts, which was a real treat, and he got to interact with kids much different from him. He had become friends with the neighbor's son, Josh Illsley and the adventures began. They were inseparable and are still extremely close to this day. Some of our friends used to call them Salt and Pepper, referring to the fact that Josh was white and Homer was black, but that did not make any difference at all. They were just Homer and Josh.

His only problem up here was that he was the only black person in town and he used to come home and say, "People keep staring at me, and the girls wanted to touch my hair." I am sure they were staring at him, as anyone can agree that when someone is staring at you, you tend to know. I explained it to him that if there was a room full of white rabbits and someone put a black rabbit in the group, which one would you see first and follow? He got it, and all was good in Homerville. One of my favorite memories was when he was exploring the property, and Josh's family used to pasture their cows on our property. One day he went down and mingled with them. I was working on the hill above and suddenly saw him running, and then the cows stampeding behind. I called out to him and asked him what he was doing. He said he was chasing the cows. I simply asked, "If you are chasing them, why are they behind you?" There was no reply.

Homer loved swimming. He would swim in the small river behind the house, and I would take him to a historical site he loved called the Floating Bridge, to swim and fish. I would pick him up, and he would always want to stay longer. He became well known to the locals. Three, four and five times I would go, and that got old. I decided to dig a pond on the property where he could just roll out of bed and jump in with a Tarzan swing and dock. He had no idea I was doing it. Every pond should have a name, so I decided to call it Homer's Pond. It was identified with a sign made by a good friend who had a sign company, Paul Margison. The day he came up, it was swimming all day while biking and playing sports the rest of the time, usually with Josh. If you saw Josh, Homer was not far behind, and vice versa.

We became closer and closer, but when Burt retired it was like a void. Homer stayed in Yonkers as he had a lot of close ties and family and I didn't see or hear from him for some time. Burt was sick and getting worse. I knew Homer hated hospitals and would avoid them at all costs, and it was what it was. He wanted to remember Burt the way he was, and had a hard time even with his mother until she died. When Burt died, I believe that Homer's sense of loss was deeper than anyone could know. After he died, I was not going to be able to keep the house as even though I was on the deed, Burt had the mortgage, and the mortgage payments went from $2200 a month to $3600 a month. I found out later that if I had sent one penny in a check that had my name on it to the mortgage company, it would have been an indication that I was assuming the mortgage and I would be responsible. Luckily, I did not. In the end they sent me a bill saying that if I paid $478,000, the house would be mine. The beginning mortgage was less than $200,000.

During that time Homer moved up and stayed with me, and helped me when I bought a new house. He was such a great support and assisted me moving in. It was a real bonding time. We were sleeping in recliners side by side in the TV room, as the house needed a ton of renovations. It was good to have him there through all this. Now he has his own room which he uses when he is up here, and with all the pictures of him in the room that I took over the years, he can now see how wonderful his life really was. I am so proud of him, and I know he still has anger issues and is struggling in many ways to be the person he wants to be and have the job he wants to have. Yet he has many barriers that are in his head only. I understand that as I too have struggled (and still struggle) to succeed. I have many mentors, and Homer is one of them. I cannot lead his life for him, and he has to take responsibility for who he is and what he does. He is an amazing person who grew up in two worlds: the housing projects, which were mostly black, poor, and drug infested, and the rectory, a sanctuary where he was surrounded by so many diverse cultures and people, but mostly white. I remember him saying to someone that he did not want anyone to know where he lived, as it would label him in some way. He was a smart cookie, and even though he is in his 30s, I still call him Kiddo.

So that young, struggling, confused young boy became an amazing, talented, and smart young man who I respect and cherish as my son. So thank you, Homer, for showing me how to be the father I never knew I could be, and tolerating the learning sessions for both of us. And thank you for giving me a granddaughter and grandson. The legacy continues. Love you, Kiddo.

To close this chapter, I just want to say that if you see some injustice or a person who could use some mentoring, introduce yourself. Do not take it over; Let it grow on you. Be sincere about who you are and learn to take the ups and downs with a vision of what could be, and not of what just happened. It may not work out the way you want or think it should, but at some point you can look back on it and know you tried to make a difference. And remember that it is a two-way street, or one hand washes the other.

One other thing - throughout my life I have learned that injustice, racism, segregation, prejudice, and hate are all learned characteristics. Many times, I see a kid who may say something racist or unjust, and I can say to myself, "I know where that comes from." When I meet someone or see something on TV that is hateful, I think to myself, "I wonder where that came from." It must come from somewhere in someone's life. It had to be learned, so someone or something had to teach them it was okay. In our society we look back at the history of racism, and we can see where a lot of it came from. I look at myself when something bubbles up and I try to find where that came from in my past. There is always a place where it must have originated.

ALL JUICED UP

In early 2001 while working for the school system, I noticed a change in my walk and my knees were in a bit of pain. Just walking from class to class was a minor challenge. I decided to go to the doctor and see what was up and he felt I needed to see a specialist, so I did. Long story short, he told me I might need an operation on at least one, if not both of my knees. You can imagine what went through my mind. I liked skiing, hiking, and biking, and I was not about to change that. Also, a long recovery, a lot of pain and loss of work, and never mind the cost, was not something I was going to look forward to.

Of course, I was polite when I told him, "Over my dead body!" I went home with a lot of questions and a lot of decisions to make. I had been on a vitamin supplement regime to stay as healthy as I could and keep my energy up. For several weeks, I dealt with the pain and each day my knees seemed to get worse.

I had seen an advertisement on TV about healthy eating and making juice from vegetables and fruits. I was intrigued by this and wondered if it was for me. The "self Caregiver" in me was showing. I quickly got on my computer, which I had recently learned how to navigate. It was one of those monsters and took forever to boot up through the phone. I typed in the search box knees, knee injuries, and fruits and vegetables that would help with my knee joints. I read article after article, and this went on for weeks.

What I found was that celery kept coming up, but more often, pineapple and grapefruit popped up as superfoods for knees and joints in general.

I had to juice the pineapple with the skin on and peel the grapefruit but use the white pulp and core. Now to get a real juicer to finish the job. Jack LaLanne had juicers I had seen on TV, and it seemed like the answer (if you ever underestimated the power of advertising, believe me, it worked).

I went out and got my first juicer. I was psyched and could not wait. I learned later was that at the thrift shop you can find a juicer in good condition for $10 or so as opposed to $150 to $300 new. Most people do not like the work it takes to clean up every time, so they use it a few times and then donate it. I have seven of them in case I need parts, or one breaks down. I felt like a professional juicer. I started drinking two glasses a day. For a while it was okay, and I could see changes, but it got old fast and it took time to do it every day. I began to make a weekly gallon and kept it in the fridge. One glass a day became the norm. With all the fruit and vegetable juice I was making and drinking, I began to feel great and energized. It gave me more vitality and strength than I had felt in quite a while.

Six months went by and I was due for another visit to the doctor, but before I went I needed a blood test, an x-ray of my knees and a stress test. Finally, I got to see the doctor. He came into the room with a curious look, but I was ready for anything he had to say. I felt I had done all I could do on my side. He sat down and said, "I have good news and bad news. The good news is that you do not need an operation. The bad news is, I don't know why." We discussed what I had been doing with the juice and he shrugged his shoulders and said, "Keep doing what you are doing." So, I have. My knees are fine 17 years later, and I have learned so much about healthy eating and how it makes me feel healthier and younger.

I have expanded into more vegetables and watch what meats I eat, which has been a life-changing experience. If you are wondering what this has to do with caregiving, well as far as myself is concerned, if I don't take care of myself, I cannot take care of others. It also has been something I can share with many people who have cancer and a lot of the people I work with.

One of the juices I shared the most (and mind you, you may have to acquire a taste for it) is a vegetable combination. I call it my blood injection because of the color the beets give it.

Four or more beets
One or two packages of celery, or about thirty stalks
Two cucumbers, or more if you like
One head of cauliflower
Three heads of broccoli
Four red peppers, not hot unless you like them hot
Twenty carrots
Four, five, or more apples for sweetness, and lately I am using at least eight

I strain it all through cheesecloth into a gallon jug and put it in the fridge so I can have a couple of glasses a day without as much work. Many of these veggies are cancer fighters and help with digestion, liver, and bowel support. It is a win-win situation.

Oh yeah, there is a mess, but I also found that if I save the vegetable pulp and freeze it as I can use it in soups or make carrot cake or zucchini bread. Some people I know make pancakes out of them for breakfast. That one I need to look up. Many things can be done with the pulp to create a healthy diet, but the main thing is to keep yourself in tip-top fitness, and you too can be all juiced up.

A New Adventure

I had been working at a small Vermont School for about fourteen years and began to find myself at that point where I felt like I had been there too long. I had a great rapport with the students, and still do. There was a dramatic change in administration, and in most cases that can only mean some turmoil. I had been working with some of the more challenging students. These are the students who teachers would prefer not to deal with in the classroom because it takes energy and attention away from the students who are there to learn. I presume I was successful, as I was increasingly asked to work with more and more students who were, for many reasons, not classroom material, and I mean that in the most compassionate way. Most of them had some form of learning disability. Some had been charged with some infraction and were suspended, which meant I was to work with them in an office in the administration building, away from other student distractions. When one's life might be challenged by events and individuals, in their out of school life, it can totally consume and divert their attention away from the "normal" educational process. It becomes difficult to act or present themselves in a way that is conducive to learning the way we know it.

I was asked by a coworker one day, "How do you work with these kids so successfully?" My answer was simple. I listen. I listen to their joys and hates. I listen to who they are and let them know that I am listening, but also find out what their passion is. By learning what that is, I can pull them in whenever I want. By letting them know that some of their inappropriate behavior is just that, inappropriate, I let them know in a way that does not make them wrong. It becomes a discussion rather than a penalty. I sometimes let them put one over on me, and I laugh along with them. I do this until they trust me, and then we start to work.

At this point, I would let them know the rules about drugs, as a few of the kids I dealt with were smoking pot or using other drugs. If I was unsure if they were using or not, I would still let them know, just in case. I would say to them, "If you smoke pot, I want you to be safe, so if you come in high I want you to give me a one to five rating of how high you are. One being fine or drug free, and five being you need to go home." If they had pot on them for whatever reason, like they forgot it was in their pocket, I told them to tell me they need to visit their grandmother, meaning "Take me home so I can dispose of it." They would never have to tell me they had a joint on them, but it gave them a chance to correct the situation. Believe it or not, it worked. Most of them eventually returned to the classroom in some form, and for the most part they were drug free, at least during school. This was a very small percentage of the kids I worked with. I found that when I used a process called harm reduction, which was used widely in the substance abuse field when I was working in NYC. This is where we work with the student, client, or person using. The idea behind it is specifically to take steps to reduce the risk of harm if a person decides to use instead of punishing them for their addiction. A school that doesn't practice harm reduction would take away the pot, and maybe even call the police. It slowly allows them to take control of the process of going to work, school or program, drug-free. It is never 100% successful, but I have seen where it works and has been able to at least gain the trust of so many students who normally would not budge. Unfortunately, with the rules in the schools becoming stricter and with all the shootings happening, harm reduction is not workable in the education system.

At any rate most, if not all of them, still keep in touch with me, and I have been to several weddings, which says a lot. Most are in their 20s and 30s, and have become great friends of mine. Some even have come over for the weekend to help renovate my house. There were a lot of naysayers concerning my methods of working with these kids. Many of my coworkers were just out of college, and I fear that there is not much education concerning street smarts or working with kids who must go back to their problems after a day at school and come back in the morning and start over again. Groundhog's Day all over again. Unfortunately, they had the degree and I didn't, and at one point was put on probation because I refused to make some statements to a student, which, if said to me, would have been insulting.

Summer vacation came and went and school began again in September. I still felt uneasy about my job situation, but felt I needed to stick to it. I did not want to let the kids down. My biggest support was the janitor who was the union steward and had to be at several meetings. He later told me he could not understand why I did not protest more against my interrogators, which is what I felt like doing. It has been my experience that protesting would do more harm than good, and letting them think they won this one was better than a suspension.

I was lucky enough to have been offered a job at another school further north by someone who knew me and knew my work. When I gave my notice after working fourteen years there, no one believed me. That was partly because I would idly threaten to leave sometimes when the pressure was on. I also acknowledged that I am not perfect and I did things that many hardened teachers would not agree with, but I knew how vulnerable these kids were at times and went to bat for as many as possible to get them through what was described to me as "high school hell" by some of the students. Most of these kids have turned out fine and are married with their own kids and great jobs. I am not saying that they did not do anything wrong; they did in many cases. When I dealt with them as students who were broken in some ways and showed them that they can get through this, it worked, and I was able to reintroduce them to the classroom. Many had to somehow realize that it was not the end of the world. I sometimes wonder what I would do if I were a student in this day and age of technology, social networks, bullying and so much information we are jamming down their throats they are hurting.

Sympathetic to what I had gone through, my friend, who had been my supervisor at one time, helped me decide to leave. The school hired me after several interviews. I again was introduced to kids who were not classroom material or had physical or mental disabilities that interrupted their educational success. I was in my element again, and had permission to explore the possibilities.

Life was good and yet I knew that the few people who did not like me or how I approached things were going to make things difficult. So, I was transferred to a program out of the school that dealt with the most difficult kids in the school. A match made in heaven. Again, I found that people did not agree with my philosophy, even if I was making pathways for so many kids. The director of that program did not want to see me go, but the decision came down from above. I never figured out why the kids felt so safe with me, but I think it might have been my calmness and ability to listen without judging.

The trade school, attached to the high school, was looking for someone who could go from student to student and make sure they were on track. I had developed a reputation of being able to calm the unruliest, and I had a great rapport with the teachers there. I had about six students that I would check in on during the day. I became that part of their day that they would wait for, because I praised them for the good work they were doing and always asked if they needed any help with anything. We would also joke a lot to lighten up the situation, and sometimes, we had a contest going where we would see who had the best appropriate jokes. Sometimes I wish I had recorded them as they were quite creative and they had to make them up themselves. But mostly, I let them teach me how to teach them.

After about a year of working there, I started volunteering for ReSource, a nonprofit organization that was based on a philosophy of recycling the things that people could no longer use any more. People would drop items off, then volunteers would check them out and anything that was not sellable would be recycled, such as electronics, metal, and wood. Anything that could be sold was put on display in this old granite shed, which was enormous. The money received would pay for employees, maintenance of the building which was heated by a pellet and electricity by solar. The building was so tight there was very little loss of heat. The rest of the money was used to fund a volunteer program to help the community with their diversion programs, and parole requirements to volunteer for an organization as well as educate them so they could successfully get jobs. It also funded a few programs to give young people a final chance to get their diploma and learn a trade. I found it to be very successful, and well run, I might add.

While volunteering there, I was asked if I wanted to work for them. I kept putting it off because I loved working with the kids in school, even though the pay was lousy. I told them I would think about it and kept saying, make it worth my while and I will consider it. I saw such an opportunity there to use all the talents I had learned throughout life, retail, management, volunteerism, nonprofit, teaching, and my love for antiques and design. They also had a platform that was raised to the ceiling, and when lowered it became a stage where we could have concerts and entertainment. It was called the Flying Stage. My experience in the theater was going to come in handy. I was finally offered a position I could not refuse. I would become the manager of this location, and would have the opportunity to transform this pile of great stuff into a well-organized retail establishment.

The problem again was the fact that I had to leave the kids. It was my first love, but I had to make a decision. I decided to let them in on it and let them help me decide. Amazingly, it worked. I had helped them so much that they wanted me to be happy. Every one of them gave me a letter to take with me and have forever. I have a folder with over 200 letters from students in the school who felt that I made a difference in their lives.

I spent a year there and worked with the Flying Stage program, which was amazing. All the merchandise and display units were on wheels and were moved off the main floor to make way for the audience. There was a lot of push back due to personality conflicts, politics, and the fact that it was a lot of volunteer work. The commitment was not there, mostly because of the logistics, and unfortunately it was stopped after I left, for a lack of funds to continue my position.

One door closes, and another door opens, and I now work with the local mental health program and work as a One on One (meaning one adult with one client) and am still a PCA for my friend Nate who I have been with now 22 years.

It is OK to be true to who you are and what you believe in. Even if there are people who want to pull you down for whatever reason, you must stand up for yourself and do what you believe is right, even if it costs you your job. After I lost my job of a lifetime, I hit rock bottom emotionally and found that place called depression. What I also found was that the depression was mine and the world was business as usual, no matter how mad I was. I was talking to a friend of mine (Bogdan, from Ukraine) and he was telling me that a co-worker was trying to make him look bad to his boss. We had a long conversation about it, and because he is in the software industry, I assumed they were both about the same age. Turns out my friend is about 26 and the guy who wants him out is 55. I told my friend that 'this guy is possibly threatened by you because you, at 26, have worked with computers all your life and know a lot about it'. He is 55 and has a time limit and an age factor if he loses his job, he may not be in the running, because companies want young people they can nurture and help grow with the company.

My friend had not considered that and thanked me for that point of view, since he wanted to talk to his boss. Now he could use a more compassionate approach to the conversation, which would be better than any accusations. I have found that in most cases, not understanding where the other person is coming from and who they are as a person can be detrimental to a situation. I have learned so many techniques while working with students who come from a place I could never understand unless I went through it. Trying to get a glimpse of that place is imperative to resolving any conflict and can soften the toughness of the situation. I still am struggling with situations where there is conflict and I have not found the right way to correct it. That will come in time. But what came out of this conversation for me was that I was 70 and I realized my depression came from my fear of being too old. Yet I was lucky to have landed the jobs I have now, and am grateful for having them.

In the caregiving world this is vital, as knowing what the person is going through or where they come from can make the difference between a successful adventure and a disaster. For instance, knowing that a person was active most of their life and now is bed-bound most of the time, as I found with Frank and Elsie, can change the approach to the relationship. Showing some compassion about the challenges they may be going through can help the interactions work successfully.

Any new adventure, no matter what it is, can be subject to this type of understanding. to know whether people are with you and how you can be the difference between enjoying your job and leaving it can be vital.

Walt Disney used to stand in line as a tourist and listen to the customers. I did this in ReSource, as well as in the school in different ways. It gave me a glimpse of how the customers viewed what I was doing and if it was working. Customers not knowing I was the manager allowed me to make comments and see what the response was. It was a key tool to put the customers needs and wants first. Keep your mind open in every situation you are in, and you will find that the world can be your mentor.

Never be afraid to start a new adventure. If you look at it and dissect it so you understand it, and it fits who you are, go for it. There is my granddad again. Life is so short, and as I get older I realize that more and more, and I am willing to start new adventures all the time. I like doing this especially when people say to me, "Sell the 16 room Victorian and retire and find an apartment that you do not have to care for." "Care for" is the key phrase. I am a Caregiver by nature and if I were not true to my nature I would just fade and die. I know that now after my four-month depression. I got a glimpse of who I was when I was not a Caregiver. It was not pretty. I thank my friend Alex for taking me out for beers and seeing the truth. His support and friendship were just what the doctor ordered. He saved my life in some ways, and we try to meet up once a month for that beer or two and good company. Sometimes we need to be cared for and must allow that to happen. Listen to your peers, and you will see a perspective of who you are that you may not see yourself. It can help you with your legacy and how life treats you, or how you treat life.

Legacy shows up in so many ways. Two of my best friends came to my aid when I was scheduled for an operation on my foot. Joe and Jami met each other at Camp Happyness and have been two of my closest friends for the last fifty years. I was to undergo surgery and was looking for someone to take me to the hospital and then back home. Now Joe and Jami live in Rhode Island, and I live in Vermont, About a four-hour drive. I had posted on my Facebook page that I needed a ride. No sooner had I posted it did I receive a response that they would do it. They came up, took me to the hospital, waited till it was done, took me home, and went back to RI. Joe at the time was battling cancer and was about to undergo treatment. This is what happens when the legacy you leave is a good one. I cannot thank them enough, and want them to know they are like family to me.

Enjoy your new adventures. I am looking for mine as I write and you read. I have to say that this book has been one of the most amazing adventures I have ever had. I recommend it to anyone. This book is also a testament to my love for new adventures. From the camps I founded or worked with, my photography, work in theatre, travel, nonprofits and school experience, they have all brought me to this point in my life. May you all have that experience in your life and share what you know with the next generation even if it is only with your kids. That will be your legacy.

HOSPICE

The dictionary tells us that it is a home or unit providing care for the terminally ill. Is that not what a hospital does?

In the mid-nineties, the ignorance and fear that plagued the AIDS population was wide-spread. Many of the hospital workers were frustrated and afraid to work in the units where there was reportedly an AIDS patient. I experienced this in 92 when Mark was admitted for the last time. I only wished that Hospice had been more prevalent and better understood before he died, although he was well taken care of by a select few nurses who refused to wear the helmets that had a plastic shield for the face that was "required" by most staff.

After Mark died, I was lost emotionally but interested in doing something to change the stigma and professional attitude of the staff in hospitals. That was when I began to hear more about the world of Hospice. I heard through the grapevine that there was a new revolution happening in New York concerning hospice. It was something that would change how we take care of all people with terminal diseases in the future.

The changes I was seeing were a welcome sight. Imagine, treating human beings humanely. To make one's life a joy rather a tragedy in the end. To live your last days with the people around you who were not afraid to touch or hug you. Wow! Now, also called Palliative care as well as Hospice, it was one of the most remarkable changes in health care in years and would change the face of care professionally as well as with families.

I had volunteered to help in a hospice in NYC for a little while and found that something that was normal to me and the right thing to do was such a novelty. The New documentary "5B" produced by Dan Krauss and Paul Haggis is such a good example of how it was and how it has changed the way we care for people with terminal illnesses. Just in the last 30+ years we have gone from one hospice to about 5,000 across the US. I feel proud and lucky to have witnessed and experienced it first hand and to have been a part of it. Another film which I believe I mentioned earlier in this book, is called, One Foot on a Banana Peel, One Foot in the Grave, Director: Johnathan Demi and staring, Juan Botas, and Lucas Platt.

Though my experience with Hospice is limited, the time I spent with them was amazing. I was so used to having nurses come in to work with Burt. When Hospice came in it was a whole different story. They were not so much interested in his being well but more interested in his well-being. I would come home early and find them all laughing and cracking jokes, eating dips and crackers, exchanging recipes and talking about books. He would be out on the deck or in the yard. It was all about feeling good, not better.

What changed for me was my stress level went way down. I was not so depressed and when I came home, we had a lot more to talk about. It was not just what he had seen on TV, it was what happened and who came over. To be honest, I think he lived an extra year or two because of the support of Hospice. What Hospice did for the success of patients and increasing their quality of life was remarkable.

Hospice

From darkness to light
From fear to calm

My days are short
So they tell me

The uncertainty of knowing when
Plagues my mind

Sometimes only I can feel
But not express

I see through the smiles and laughter

Lets make him as comfortable as possible

How do you comfort my soul

My fear sleeps with me each night
Poking my dream state with a cry

The 'why me' comes out at night
That's where I hide

Yet when I awake
Your smiles make the fear seem far away

Your comforting hands and words
Carry me through the day's challenges

Making me feel wanted
Needed
Not alone

Yet this is where the fear of legacy
Peeks in the door

What legacy swill I leave?

What do and will they think of me

I make a list of what I have done
Some good
Some not so good

I have cursed at some
Because I was afraid

I have slandered others
Even if only in my thoughts

Yet I have led
A kind and compassionate life

And then I think to myself
Who the hell cares?

What does it matter?

I will be gone.
They will forget the me I have left with them

And again I feel the palliative or soothing
Voices of the humans, heroes, who are with me now

I realize,
I cannot change the past
Or regulate, with precision, the future

All I have is now
And
Hospice is my strength
My glue
My oxygen

So,
I surrender to the now
With my hospice family

By Eli Shaw

TIDBITS

The most difficult thing for the human mind to comprehend or deal with is the experience of not knowing, is not knowing what we don't know. We know what we know, but when we don't know something, this is when it becomes an impossible task and incomprehensible. When we are in the middle of our ignorance and bliss occurs, we don't know what we don't know, but when we realize we know we don't know, that's when the bliss dissipates, and the adrenaline can flow. As I said earlier, everyone is ignorant of everything at some point in their life. We must learn everything we know, and must know that we will always be ignorant about something as long as we are conscious.

Complacency

The sad part of curing a disease or getting a disease manageable is that we no longer take the disease seriously. When HIV and AIDS were considered a death sentence people were more focused on prevention, its causes, and how to lead a fuller life while they were alive. When sustainable drugs were introduced, that focus and passion for succeeding would slow down.

When drugs were introduced to help keep the illness or virus sustainable and help people lead a fuller and longer life, many people did not take precautions or use protection, and did not take the illness seriously. The reason being that if they contract the virus, there is something they can take to keep them alive, and if they did get it, you're almost guaranteed a fuller and longer life, compared to the early years because of the medications they could take.

Attitude

I have come to believe that of all the ailments a person can have, or contract with all the billions of personality traits there are in all the different cultures the one thing I find that is the hardest to overcome, for many reasons, is a bad or unjust attitude. The only cure comes from within, and this is the hardest thing to treat because many of us cannot let things go. We mill them around in our minds and try to justify why we are or have been hurt, bullied or unjustly treated. We eventually carry it around so much that it will affect every inch of our existence. We share our distaste with people we meet, and it becomes viral. I have seen this in many instances with some who take their anger from having the disease and what it has done to their lives and place it in the laps of people they care about. I did this when I went through my depression after being let go from the one job I loved the most. It was not until I heard the phrase "Let it go," and people not wanting to hang with me as I was so angry that I began to look at that option. Letting go was hard. I had to go deep into myself and pull up all the courage I could muster to heal and move on.

Endurance

Someone asked me once, "How do you handle being a Caregiver every day with so many emotions on both sides of the fence?" I had to think about this one a lot and realized that whenever I went into the room no matter what mood I was in or what had happened to me before, I had to walk in with a great attitude and a smile and not let the person's sadness affect me. If I went in with a bad attitude or was angry, I could not take care of the person as well as I should, especially if it was compounded with their anger. If I went in with an amazing attitude, I could handle anything. It is not an easy thing to do. I see it with nurses when they enter a new patient's room after something bad has happened and they have a smile on their face and a caring presence. I have also seen the negative side of that with nurses, and all you get is a dissatisfied consumer (patient or client receiving services) who will pass it on even further. I found I had to do it a lot before it was natural for me. When I am with Nate, I am often smiling and joking, and he is now so glad to see me, and it becomes a wonderful encounter. Humor is one of the best remedies, even if it is a bad joke. Believe me, it works.

Listen

Listen to everyone you work with or for. Get all the information you can about who they are, their needs, their passions, and their dreams. You will find that having that knowledge will allow you to be successful with anything you do.

Laugh

Laughter is one of the best cures for depression, sadness, illness and just a bad hair day. Stand in front of a mirror when you are upset and look at yourself. Now smile. Keep smiling and see how those muscles can transform your brain cells to make you believe that things are okay. When we only see ourselves from the inside we lose sight of the big picture and how others perceive us. It is like having a bad hair day. If you cannot see what you look like, you can't change it.

Believe

Believe in something. Believe in nature, the warmth of the sun, the coldness of the snow, or the strength of the wind. Things that are real or tangible are the easiest things to believe in. It is the intangible things that can be elusive. If nothing else, believe in yourself. If you pinch yourself, you will know you are real.

Breathe

Take time to breathe. Breathe slowly. Breathe consciously. Breathe in and know that it is good. By doing so, you will find a peace that will heal you. Our breathing is so often trapped in our daily events and unconsciously patterns our stress or activity. For example, when we panic, our breathing goes faster, when we relaxed it goes slower, when we exercise we breathe to the beat of what we are doing, and it is all unconscious. When we become conscious of it, there is a sense of control that we sometimes lose as we move throughout the day. This control can change our attitude and health.

Protection

I have recently been seeing advertisements on TV about getting tested not just for HIV/AIDS, but for so many other STDs. It has been over 35 years since the first cases of HIV/AIDS were diagnosed. At that time, it was a death sentence. I remember meeting someone who mentioned that he had the virus. I knew his mother at work, and when she found out, she knew it would not be long before she would have to bury him. She was right. It was only a few months before he began to look like a walking skeleton. I felt bad for his mother.

After he died, she began a one-woman campaign to get everyone she thought could be at risk to get tested. Most of them just said, "why should I get tested? I would rather not know and just die then go around for months knowing I am going to die." This was a common sentiment. Also, the importance of condom use after the as protection after the sexual revolution of the 60's was a message that was slowly getting out. We did not know that much about the virus yet so it was a tough sell. This went on for years and to be honest, one of the biggest problems with the virus was that if you contracted it once, you had a better chance of living longer. You were still going to die, but you could live a longer life. There are people out there who have had the virus since the 90s and are still alive because they got infected only once. The problem arises when you get infected multiple times. Each time you have sex with someone with HIV you receive the virus again. Instead of the virus multiplying, you multiply the times you got infected which usually leads to an early and painful death.

For many years it was well-received that using condoms and getting tested was the only defense against a quick death sentence. Now more than 35 years have passed, and the death count worldwide is in the millions, as many were not documented as AIDS-related. We are still pushing campaigns about safe sex and getting tested. We have become complacent. People are still getting infected, but the difference is the medication has advanced so much that they can live a full and productive life. This means that people are lax as far as the fear of getting infected. We are over the era of tallying up the numbers and publishing the flyers that tell you what a death sentence it is.

We still need to be aware of who our partners are and how to be safe. If you have had any risky or unprotected sex with someone you do not know the history of, you need to get tested. There have been many people who said, "Well, I have been in a relationship for many years. I don't have to worry." Unfortunately, that is not a sure thing. It was not then, and it is not now. Today with the of drugs that can keep the virus under control, the fact that this virus is still around means it is still a risk.

Another problem is that kids or teens are having sex earlier and more frequently than before. Remember when you were young and foolish? Teens think they know better as usual, and even though we have very comprehensive educational tools in place in school, not all of them are listening. Their hormones are a stronger influence. The one sure thing is that if you have not had sex ever, you are fine. The virgins win this time.

So, get tested, use a condom, openly ask your partner if they have been tested, and practiced safe sex. Remember, oral sex is not safe sex.

Looking for Passion

After being a Caregiver for so many years, I found that in every case, finding the passion and history of the person you are caring for can open the door to success. There have been situations where the person being cared for was in a slump or depression, which can be devastating. When I was going through depression, I was falling deeper and deeper with nothing to grab onto. Things I could have done while being without a job that would have pulled me out of that deep depressing hole seemed so far away and almost inaccessible until a friend of mine came by and knew what would make my day. It was only a moment compared to the length of time I was depressed, but it was a door that I could either close or keep open. it is my choice.

Working as a Caregiver, it is so important to make sure you have some doors you can show them that will take them out of the slump, or just away for a while. With Nate, who is pretty much bed bound, I would just put him into a wheelchair and take a walk around the block, or put headphones on him and play Woods Tea Company, Queen, or Gregorian chant music, which he loved. Go figure, but it took his mind away from the pain of the situation. Humor is another way. He loves when I fall or bump into something, on purpose.

Knowing the things people like or the things that calm them is so important. If you are just guessing, then put yourself in a situation where someone was trying to calm you down in a situation you felt uncomfortable in. Communication, is critical to a successful caregiving relationship. Just ask, and you might be surprised. I have been working with Nate for over 22 years, and I know pretty much everything he likes and dislikes. It was hard in the beginning, as he was nonverbal. I had to watch his reactions to sounds, music, and visuals. It took a long time. When I was working with people who could discuss it with me, it has been a bit easier, but the key is to remember what they say or express and watch their reactions.

When working with teenagers, finding out what their passion is can be the difference between a good teacher/student relationship or a disaster. Every student I worked with, I spent a lot of time in the beginning getting to know them, who they are, what they like, and what they do not like in regards to music, cars, sports, and food. It all came in handy in negative situations. I could create a diversion or distraction that would launch them out of the bad situation they were in. Granted, this usually can only happen in a one on one situation, but there are ways to do this with a class, as I watched many teachers do. Showing a movie once every two weeks that they picked off of a list can make the difference between a stressful week and one that went well.

Just remember to look for the passion, and you will be fine.

This next piece was a post from a woman I know who has three boys who I worked with in school. Suffering from depression, she knows how to express herself in the word. She sent me this to add to the book.

Depression

"Thought of the day on depression: Depression is the ability to cheer up others and make them realize how lucky they may be and how loved they are. All the while, not being able to see these same things in your own life. Encouraging others to live, while only hanging on by a small thread yourself. Outwardly, everyone thinks you're fine. When people ask how you are doing, you give an upbeat answer, as we have been conditioned to do. Suicide should not be viewed as selfish, quite the contrary. Most people who consider suicide, believe that they have nothing good to contribute to others and society and that life is more difficult to participate in that most can ever comprehend."

My dear friend,
Jolene Scott

Stroke,

Stroke, Stroke, Stroke, sounds like the rowing team in college. It's not, it is the butt end of a joke. Around 1995 I was introduced to a man who was an icon in his community. His rapport with kids in school, people in the church, and people on the street was flawless. His humor, he would say, was the only thing that would convince him that life was good, and that we were living in amazing times.

When I met him, he had just suffered a stroke. I got to know him through the many people who told stories about him. His legacy was amazing. I did not meet one person who had a bad word about him. Now he just sat there with his stricken face with a half-smile, and little control of his arms. He tried to explain to me how it felt to be him. He said, "It feels like someone had taped or glued my arms to my side, my legs together and put tape on my mouth. Now they want me to ride a bike and continue as usual." That was a visual I would not forget. His words were slurred, and yet I understood him. I could see his frustration and pain while he was talking.

I spent a lot of time with him. He taught me so much about life. He once said that I seemed to have learned a lot, and remembered almost everything he said. He also said it was not because he was a good teacher; it was because he had the patience of a saint. When he passed away, his wife told me that I was one of the only people who would visit, and she appreciated that but could not understand why, since I did not know him and he supposedly had many friends. I assume that most of the people who knew him wanted to remember him the way he was, and it was too hard for them to see him this way. For me, it was a new adventure and a way to learn more about things like this, and to meet someone truly amazing.

Fast forward about thirteen years. I got up one morning earlier than usual, and my side was numb. I thought I just slept on the wrong side, so I rolled over and went back to sleep. When I woke up to the alarm, I found that it was worse, so I slid out of bed and fell to the floor. Not knowing what was going on, I slid down the stairs and to the bathroom and got dressed. I was able to hobble to the door and to the car. Burt was still sleeping, and I felt I had to get to school as I would be late. Using my left foot and hand, I drove down the street. I noticed my face was limp on one side and decided to go to the emergency room. As I hobbled in, one of the nurses got me in a wheelchair. After a while, I began to realize it was serious. The doctor said things like "Bell's Palsy" and "stroke". I cannot tell you what that felt like, as it was indescribable. But remembering my friend from thirteen years ago, I began to make jokes.

A long story short, I had suffered some sort of damage to the base of the brain stem and top of my spine from some pressure or bump to the back of my neck, which I have never understood and never asked about, but the stroke I had was very recoverable. They also called it a transient ischemic attack which is like a warning stroke. I have now only a few residual effects from that time. One of them is from taking kindling wood and breaking it over the front of my upper leg.

It damaged the nerves, but because I could not feel my leg, I did not know it was damaging them. Duh! Not the smartest thing I have ever done. I also have a twitch in my face and eye at times, but for the most part I had a complete recovery. The thing that pulled me through was my persistence and commitment to getting the feeling on my right side back. I found an old massage vibrator in a box. I started to use it on my arms and legs to see if that helped. When I went to the doctor a few months later, he was amazed at my progress.

Friends did not come by often and except for the loyal few, I seldom saw people. I admit that I was focused on my health, but it would have been nice. The other thing that bothered me was that some people at work were saying I was faking, as no one heals that quickly from a stroke. Ta da, yes, they do. It all depends on where, how, and what kind of a stroke it is. I think that was the most frustrating thing to me, that they did not believe me. The thing that pulled me through was definitely my humor, and remembering what my friend from the 90s taught me. I have to say it was a difficult adjustment, and it does feel like someone has tapped your leg and arm down. But thank God my mind was still in tact and my will and my friends who were there for me from all over and especially on Facebook were there for me. It wasn't all bad.

Five years later, I lost my finger to a saw, and a few years after that I lost Burt. It was a bad run, but I kept my chin up and laughed and smiled. That joke about strokes? "What do you call it when the college rowing team has a stroke epidemic?" I did not say it was a great joke, but coming from my old friend with the stroke it was hilarious. Just remember how much you can learn from everyone you meet, even the ones you don't like or care for. Especially the ones who tell bad jokes.

Quality of care

Many years ago, while working with some residents in the Group Home in Andover for people with disabilities, I began questioning myself about my quality as a Caregiver and what I was doing to make their lives better. In many cases, I saw I was trying too hard to make their lives more comfortable, and in exchange I was not comfortable or satisfied with what I was doing and how I was doing things. One of the residents who had a TBI and was blind became one of my greatest teachers. I would try to keep him from running into things by yelling "Watch out!" or "A little to the left!" I did not realize that my directions were not helping, and usually did not mean anything to him as my perception was much different from his. What I was doing was only distracting him from succeeding, and hampering his ability to make it on his own.

One day, he decided to tell me that what I was doing was not working for him. He said, "Let me tell you what I need you to do." From that point on, I understood that what I was doing was only making me feel like I was important or had some control of the situation, and that only benefited me. There has to be an equal investment between Caregiver and one being cared for.

Here are my times when we need to have the person being cared for teach the Caregiver how best to care for them. You may say, "What if they cannot talk?" Well, if you have ever been in love and used your eyes or expression to communicate how you feel, or how much you care, you can understand how important it is to learn any way possible how to best care for someone. They can guide you. Let go of what you know and learn what you can about the person you are caring for. Also, if you are the one being cared for, the same thing applies. Learn as much about your Caregiver as you can. Let that guide you. Teach them what is best for you and what will make the most sense in your relationship. Granted, there will be times when that cannot happen because of personality clashes or different belief systems, but for the most part, it works.

As I started to work in the school system, I began to realize that this same technique is extremely valuable in the success of the student's experience with the school and with me. I would always ask them, "Teach me how to teach you." Our school or educational system is based on the assumption that the teacher knows everything and the student should do their job as a student and learn. Many times the techniques of teaching (or, like I said, personality conflicts) will get in the way, and it becomes a push and pull. This is when and why we have so many para educators and Special Ed personnel. It is a solution, but a costly one, and one that is needed with all the breakdowns in our systems. For one teacher to focus on the individual issues of so many children is not possible, and the lessons would suffer. Let them teach us how to teach them. Let them teach us how to care for them. Let them teach us, as the one being cared for, how best we can help them take care of us. Let us be open to not knowing, and admitting that we do not know how to best teach them or care for them and, please, do not feel bad that we do not know. Swallow your pride and learn about them, who they are, and what makes them tick.

What if?

Knowing what I know now about the AIDS epidemic that we experienced in the 80s and 90s, I wonder what it would be like now if it began the same way at the same magnitude with the instant gratification of the internet, social media, anonymous bullying, and the way we seem to treat each other as punching bags. Remembering many of the statements I heard from people in my travels who did not even know anyone who had the virus and the judgment that went on then, I truly believe that it would be devastating.

Patience....

A while ago, I visited the Vermont Bird Museum with my clients. It is not the usual bird museum that you would think of seeing. It is a museum that is filled with almost 500 hand carved birds found in Vermont, their sounds and history. Near the building there are trails and vantage points to see live birds in their natural habitat. These works of art are so lifelike, you could almost see them move.

The part of this tour that astounded me was that the artist, Robert Spear Jr. who is a native of Vermont and began his work at a young age. One of the birds, the full-size replica of a turkey, a gem of a tom, took over 2000 hours to create. I can only imagine the patience that this took. I split from the main group and as I was walking with my client and listening to the bird calls through the speakers, I watched his eyes light up when he saw the eagle, which is his favorite bird. Seeing this woke up another "ah-ha" moment in my mind. I saw how the work and passion of the legacy of this one man has and will spark delight and awareness in the eyes of so many.

I bring up the word patience because it is a word I have used in my work. I have had to become aware of the patience I have in my life, in my caregiving and maturing capacities. I look back at all the things I have accomplished and experienced and still don't know fully why it all happened. I am in wonder of how time can be on our side and how patience has a part in it all. Patience in the daily encounters with our clients and associates, our beliefs, and our barriers, is something that happens to all of us, but most of us are unaware. Many of us are impatient with others as well as ourselves.

I look at Mr. Spear, his talent and his passion and commitment to what he believed in and how it could be passed on to so many. His legacy was well-intentioned and quite successful, as opposed to mine which was quite haphazard and unintentional, yet my passion and commitment was the same. I felt such a kinship with this man through his art and his amazing commitment to teaching and learning. As I look at my commitment to writing this book, I have opened the gates of learning.

I did not know how to write, and sometimes feel I still don't. The difficult parts for me were receiving criticism even when it pissed me off. My patience with myself, my passion and my connections to all the people I have met through my journey has been a rough ride. Seeing how Mr. Spear pushed on from that first bird he carved to the large wooden turkey, it has helped me see clearly where I have come from, where I am, and where I want to be when it comes to this book and the patience I needed to finish it. Patience is one of the most valuable assets in the caregiving world. Without it, there would be chaos and uncertainty. If you are a Caregiver, remember that the more patient you are in dealing with clients (as you are now in their world), the more successful you will be. Time is on your side, whether you believe it or not. If you are the one being cared for, patience is key in teaching them how to care for you successfully. That relationship is also applicable to parents and kids, teachers and students, doctors and patients, and you and the people you meet each day.

This visit to the museum "Birds of Vermont" was one event in my life that happened like any other event but I was able to take from it so much that I value, and it is priceless to me. Sometimes just reading between the lines of a daily event can open up vast moments of awareness, but only if you have patience.

⬥━━━━━⬥━⬥━⬥━━━━⬥

Opportunity knocks

I had the privilege of speaking to a group of people who were extremely successful and attributed their success to just letting life guide them. Over and over I heard testimonies about the choices they made and how they came to them. They were not looking for them. One of the individuals stated the reason he believed that the opportunities kept coming to him was because of who he was and how he treated people. He is now a leading professor at a major university. He said, it allowed himself to work on who he was as a human being and how he related to others on his journey to where he sits now.

This made me think back to all the things I have done and places I have gone. They were just things or events placed in my lap because of who I was, what I was doing, and how I presented myself. I remember getting nominated for the Outstanding Young Men Of America Award and wondering why. I was not super smart, I had a low paying job, I lived in a small town, and all through my high school years I was a straight D student. I asked the guy who was presenting it to me why I got it while the mic was on, without knowing that everyone was listening. He told me it was because of my passion for justice and how I went about changing things if I found it was not agreeable. I look at the students who survived the school shootings and relate to the fact that they would not be fighting for justice and change if it had not happened. It fell into their lap, tragically. My message to them is keeping your passion in sight, but in check. Many people lose ground by forcing their passion on others and in such a partisan and tribal world we live in, accelerated by the social media phenomena, it can be explosive. We live in such a fragile society and are fragile as human beings, and that goes for the strongest of us.

What I have done in my life came from my gut. In most cases, I did not go looking for the opportunity specifically. Most of my jobs happened when I met someone and they saw something in me that they thought would benefit their cause. Even though I knew I wanted to work in design or a creative venue in retail or theater, other jobs came to me. I was thinking about what my life would have been like if I chose other avenues to work in. I thought I might do well in other fields but only saw the successes of others in that field. Not seeing the struggles they had to endure to get to be so successful, I wondered if I would I have survived. Knowing me, I am not sure I would have reached the high standards of the people I saw as success stories. I know now that my success in Caregiving was because I was being myself, and letting life happen.

In the movie *Frozen* by Disney, the song, "Let It Go" says it all to me. The ice cathedrals she created are like the programs I worked with and was able to create an amazing legacy I can now look back on. I know what it took for me to let go of what was keeping me silent or what was suppressing my passion, which was, many times, just barriers in my mind. No one else could see it until I did let it go and worked that passion openly. I am where I am because of myself, my passion, my mission, and everything around me that has happened for the past 70 years. All of these were stepping stones to the here and now.

So Blessed

I am so blessed to know that every minute of my life has been filled with excitement, challenge, wonder, fear, joy, exhilaration with the small things and ecstasy with the momentous ones, love, anger, and all the people I have met that helped me create the amazing life I have the lead and am still living. To hear a song like "Against the Wind" by Bob Seger and get that flashback rush that makes me feel that my life has been well-lived, is a joy and blessing. When I see the young people I have known, I want to somehow let them know the wonders that are out in this world and get them to look for them. I know all too well that because of the internet and social media, there is not much left in the natural world of social and experiential growth that is worthy of astonishment. It has truly been diluted. I do feel blessed.

It's Everyone's Responsibility

At Walmart I ran into an old student I had in high school. Miles Silk was one of those brilliant students who was so smart he was bored and got in trouble. He left school early until he found an alternative school, connected to his school so he could get his diploma. We had a great conversation, and when I asked him how he was doing, he said, "Just trying to pay bills and survive". One of the many things the school did not do well at was making sure the students left with a good sense of survival. I, of course, brought up the fact that the schools rely on the parents for a lot of that growth. He said, "Yeah, the school blames the parents and the parents blame the school, and the kids just don't know how important it is so they don't care."

He was right. We seem to put the blame wherever it is easiest and it has a negative affect on us. I am glad to say he is working at Walmart and paying his bills. He is now also looking into a future in writing. You can do it, Miles. It just takes a little stamina and patience, unless you are in a hurry, and then it is a crapshoot.

Holding Space

Many years ago, about 1974, I went to a retreat for people who volunteered as area representatives for foreign exchange programs. We were learning how to deal with how we interact and care for the students, who were as young as 15, while they were here under our care. It was also important for us to learn how to work with the host families during times of crisis and uncomfortable situations. One of the main concepts was to listen without judgment. This is something that we as Caregivers, parents, teachers, and people in the medical world have a hard time doing in the beginning. In our culture we are conditioned to respond, judge, and defend ourselves from childhood. It was a lesson that took me a while to understand.

Today there is a concept I have read about which has some of that in it. It is called "holding space" which to me is a much more comforting and comfortable way of saying it. We tend to judge everything. I read the article and have corresponded with the author, Heather Plett. It profoundly affected me after reading it, and I found it can be applied to anything in your life. Please allow me to share the article with you, and I thank Heather for kindly allowing me to reprint it.

Hold Space

By Heather Platt

As a bereavement support companion and someone that talks with families every day that have experienced a pregnancy or infant loss, holding space for someone is extremely vital, important and necessary. Even though I've experienced loss myself, both times being completely opposite experiences, I will never be able to experience what a family is going through that I meet. I can never compare circumstances or judge what they are going through. I can't hold expectations over them or ask them to do anything other than what they are doing. It is my place to offer love, validation, hope, and support.

Holding space for someone is not easy – we have to set aside our feelings, our hurts, our opinions, our agenda – we need to allow them to go through what they are facing at that exact moment. It's difficult for all of us to not want to voice our thoughts and feelings – but what the other person needs is space to cry, vent, yell, rationalize their own thoughts out loud. They need a safe place. A sacred space. A HEALING Embrace provides that for families. A safe place, a sacred space for families to express their deepest hurts, fears, frustration, sadness, happiness, and joy without judgement or bias opinions.

We allow families who have experienced loss to feel loved and validated, to know that they are not alone in whatever they are facing. That when the rest of the world tells them to move on or to stop hurting – we understand and allow them to feel the rawness of their story. This is a beautiful explanation of what it really means to hold space for someone. If we can all lay aside our own hearts desires and really listen to someone else – this world would be a better place.

One Last Thought

I have made many references to specific songs, music and artists who have influenced me or made a difference in my life. It is part of our nature to relate to music as hallmarks or milestones in our lives that have inspired us or it just happened to be the music of the time. In 1969 I heard a song by Reginald Dwight now known as Elton John, called Where Its At. I felt like he was singing about me.

Where It's At

Elton John
Written by Reg Dwight and Nicky James

Dada dum-da dadada dum-da
Where it's at
Dada dum-da dadada dum-da
Where it's at
He's a man who knows most everything
Of anything at all
Tells a story of psychology
And his story never falls
He's a man who wears a portobello yellow bill-bob hat
He's a man who knows exactly where it's at
He's a man who draws illusions
And he carves them on a tree
Including all the love he found
He gives to you and me
And I don't even know his name
But I surely promise that
He's a man who knows exactly where it's at
Roaming around from place to place
He takes in all that he sees
He notices the good things that please him
He...

I began to follow his work and it seemed that his songs followed me in a way. Then in the 1970s I got to see him in concert. Blew me away. He became my alter ego and gave me a voice in my head that allowed me to pull myself out of my shell of shiness. It was like his songs, creativity and flamboyant life gave me the feeling I could do anything I wanted if I just put my mind to it. I still fall back to Cat Stevens and so many other deep and meaningful artists but it was Elton who helped me grow wings. And that was before Red Bull. LOL The last song I want to hear when I die will be Song for Guy. Thanks Elton. God Bless you and your gift.

POETRY

The following poems were written by me or given to me to include in this chapter as an inspiration. Many of them could have been included in the chapters, but I thought it would be nice to keep them all together as a unit.

Janice Burns wrote a book called "Sarah's Song." When she died, I contributed this poem to the service and gave it to her relatives.

Janice's Song

There's a twinkle in the eyes of baby Sarah tonight
As her mother is coming home
To a dimension filled with grace, love, and light
In the clouds where the angels roam

The road to the gate is paved with our love
As we bid her our last good-byes
For she will be met by her loved ones above
Reunited in those heavenly skies

Complete, as she ends her short earthly stay
More complete than many I've known
Her journey is marked with love in her special way
And all she touched has grown

As she looks back on her journey, in an earthly sense
She sees our faces all aglow
She has left us a light to guide us from whence
Our hearts may continue to grow

Yes, there is a twinkle in Sarah's eyes tonight
And Bill's and St. Peter's too
For, heaven will be a place so bright
With her memories of friends like you.

So, do not be too sad that she has quietly left our side,
She was strong and she gave us her all
The memories she left with us we must not hide
These are legacies to help us walk tall

So, if on a dark night you see twinkles of light
And stars shooting across the sky
It's the angels who guide her through the dark of night
And Janice shooting home as she waves good-bye

She will be with us in thought as our tears wash away
And she talks to us while time grows long
She will also be with those she never met on the way
Through a book called Sarah's Song

So sing of her life, her teaching and her ways
Our time here is as precious as rain
And think of her kindly, remember the good days
For we too shall meet Janice again.

By Eli Shaw In memory of Janice Burns,
Author of Sara's Song, and friend

This poem was written when I found out how rich and full my life really was after spending time with a close friend who was dealing with cancer of the throat. Joe opened my eyes wider than I have ever had them with his words of memories, hopes and dreams.

Your Garden Is Full

A plot of soil, covered with weeds,
Grasses, shrubs and trees

You cleared, churned, gave nourishment
And cast the seeds you hope to reap from

As you sowed your new seeds inch by inch
Furrow by furrow

Creating an imaginary quilt
Of colors, life and nourishment

"Ah, one day I will eat the fruits
Of my labor," you say

And one day you do!

Yet there are storms to contend with
As you protect your creation

When it is dry you quench. When it is wet you
Watch that the waters do not carry it away.

Your garden is now full
And Beautiful

"Ah, with all the pain and heartache my fruits
are edible and my flowers fragrant"

*And today you absorb the nourishment long-awaited
and look upon the beauty of this garden of life.*

*For you have tended it, with the help of a force
greater than you, greater than your garden.*

*Your life is full of wisdom, and knowledge,
Based on your experiences as you make room for new seeds*

*As you remember the pain and
How painful it was then*

*You now only see the withering flowers
That has emerged out of the torrents and floods, heat and cold
As your garden has blossomed,
So do you*

*You only need to look in the reflection of another's eyes
To see your beauty as you grow within*

*And tend your garden
Whatever fruits it may bear.*

*My garden is full
And bares the fruits of love, compassion and nourishment*

*I have shared the fruits and flowers
And harvested the seeds that I shall share also*

*Look within and see your garden
It is full and your flowers fragrant*

*Your garden is full,
And the gate can always be opened to share and nourish
As I have, mine with you*

By Eli Shaw

This poem was written in response to the experience of taking in a student who had nowhere else to turn and was quite angry. Cody broke every law I laid down and rule I tried to enforce. I gave him the longest rope of compassion and acceptance, and he still had a hard time. Even though I had to tell him to leave, he and I are still in contact and close. He still takes me out to eat, but I have to pay. Today he is still angry and dealing with the law, but as we walk one step at a time, one foot in front of the other, he is alive, aware, and now has more love and compassion in his life. "Living the dream," as he frequently tells me.

A Young Angry Soul

I look at you
Your Jagger hair, rebelling against conformity

I look at your soul
Good, sincere, angry and confused

Told that your worth is less than, for so long
How can you not believe it

Told I was crazy to reach out
How could I believe that

I saw the light of the future bright
You saw the cloud of the daily effort to sustain

How can I not feel your pain
That is lashing out on my pride and soul

How can I not be angry
When you do

When I look at your face I see my past My
rebellion, my youthful arrogance

When you look at my face
I feel you see all the others
Who have failed to see your light
Yet I do, I see that light

Your ears are closed,
your mind is shut
To the wealth of knowledge waiting to invade your soul
Your eyes only see the anger,
the mistrust and rejection
Laid out before you all these years like a carpet

I do not blame you
For you

I do not expect you to be me
Or any facsimile

I only ask for your respect for what I have sacrificed
To ease your pain

I cannot save you
Yet I want to

My wish for you is for you to be rid of the pain, anger and resentment
And judge those who come along with a just and fair look

Yet I know I may be fooling myself That I believe it will come to pass

Your time is long to get where I sit And see what I have seen

Your patience, or lack of it, may overshadow that journey
Clouding any crystals that may come your way

Sit with me and let me speak
And let yourself hear what I have heard

You don't have to believe it
All I ask is that you hear it.

I too have heard many things
I did not believe
Yet I ask that you not judge me unfairly

For those wheels will surely falter and derail
The light within, within

Your doubts will guide you as they have
And your truths will push you into position

I do not share your anger
Yet I believe it to be real

I do not pretend to see the pain in your eyes,
but I know it is there

I do not hold your wishes to pretend that life is a puff of smoke

My smoke has dispersed long ago
My eyes, they are clear

And when the clear cool sensation of the liquidity of reality
Splashes your face, eyes and mind

Only then will you feel the freedom
Of whatever it is your soul is made of

Eli Shaw

During my journey between programs, caregiving situations and jobs, I found a way for kids as well as adults to express themselves with a little help. The process has to do with poetry, emotions and subjects they have a hard time talking about. It can also help them put things together. I first ask them what they want to write about. The first one called Chariot is about the wheelchair that both restricted and gave him freedom at the same time.

The second one was with Paul who has a TBI and liminited communication skills. I asked him what he wanted to write about as it was Halloween. He just started up again an exercise program on a bike and it was fresh on his mind. I asked him to give me words I could work with. The first word was bike. I asked him what color the bike was, and he said pink. He remembered the old one was not working well and said it was in a junk pile. I asked him who was riding it. He said a ghost. This went on until I had enough and we would work line by line until we had it done.

I had used this method with Portuguese Brazilians and some Japanese when I was in Brazil. It is amazing how much better they feel when they have harnessed the emotions and things that trouble them and turn it into something like a poem or a story.

This poem was written in an English Class in Whitcomb School, Bethel Vermont with my charge, Nathan Taplin who is in a wheelchair. We were to write a poem about mobility, and I helped him with the words and mood.

Chariot

The sun rises as I get
Airlifted as a rescued victim to my chariot

The shackles, keeping me safe
From the days, bumps and grinds

My dependence on this vehicle of freedom
Contradicts the world's view of the same

I sit, like a king on his throne
Shackled by responsibility

Some say he is handicapped
I say challenged

As one is challenged by his or her own weakness
I am by my lack of motion

Though I have no facility to be mobile on my own
As a horseless wagon

My reliance is profound on the strength of character
Of many to mobilize my destiny

This chariot of sorts is my ticket
To the freedom, you might take for granted

As one's feet are the vehicle to one's destination
So are the wheels of my chair

Co-writers

Nathan Taplin & Eli Shaw

This next one is Pauls. I am sure you can see what I meant about putting words together to make a story or a poem

The Halloween Bike

Each year a strange thing happens
For three hundred and sixty-four days
A very unassuming rickety old rusty bike
Sits in a junkyard, victim to the elements
But, on one very special day
October 31st to be exact
As the sun falls behind the tall pine trees in the west,
This unassuming rusty old pile of metal
Takes on a life of its own.
In the full moon light, it begins to glow and vibrate.
The rusty chips falls as the bike takes on a pinkish glow,
As if it were becoming alive.
Suddenly, as if pulled from the from the rusty pile by lightning
It hurls itself forward, down the gravel passages
between the rusty mountains of cars and refrigerators.
Suddenly it passes through the gates and into
the town glowing and vibrating.
Passing cars and up on the sidewalks,
Weaving between the pedestrians, it seems to
be leaving a trail of glowing candy.
Throughout the night, it circles the houses and trick or treaters
Spinning and swerving as if it were ridden with intention.
Some say it is ridden by the ghost of the young boy
Who owned it many years ago.
In the 1920s a young boy was hit by a runaway horse and wagon,
While riding his bike on Halloween.
He loved to throw candy from a bag while riding the streets of the town.
He would make his candy for weeks before halloween
at home and usually ran out of the red coloring.
So, the candy took on a pink glow and became his legacy.

By morning on the first of November
He passed away and his bike being unusable
ended up in the metal pile at the
Junk yard on the west side of town.
Since then, every year on that special day at sundown,
You can see a pink glow and the laughter of a
young boy, tearing through the town.

Co Writers

Paul D and Eli Shaw

Kevin was a person I met briefly after Mark had died, and he was able to give me some solid ground to stand on at the time. I never knew his last name. It is amazing to me how people can make such an enormous impact on us in such a brief time.

For Kevin

*The news of your departure brought tears and long sunken emotions
to light, I did all I could to be in control but alas, I could not fight*

*Your silence had me worried, not like you at all
With your constant support and friendship,
you pulled me through the long haul*

*After Mark passed on, you helped me laugh
And see the other side of this pandemic wrath*

*Your gentle words and uncompromising perception
Allowed me to move on in my life with an overwhelming reception*

*Your pain in life will be your salvation in death
Where your chosen loved ones await you as you took your last breath*

*Our time together on this amazing yet daunting earth
Was short and caring as we each showed our worth*

*In the silence that deafens the spirit, you suffered alone
I know your pain was more than expressed to me on the phone*

*The spirit you gave me I shall cherish and keep
In my remembrance of you, I will acknowledge
your life each night before I sleep*

So, when you get there, say hi and a big hug to all your cohorts
And one to my Mom and Dad and Mark, he's in a T-shirt and shorts

I must say goodbye or so long as I go on with
my work on this earthly realm
But remember you taught me to laugh and love
again and take my position at the helm

Goodbye my friend, don't let anyone steer you wrong
For I will see you at the gate when my time comes along

By Eli Shaw

This poem was also inspired by someone I knew who had limited mobility and how much patience I needed to understand his perspective.

My Gate

My gate, slow, precise, on purpose
The support of others essential
My world, small, yet filled with friends, close
My reliance on them evidential

You look at me with questions of how and why
I show you only what I please to
My smiles are real and laugh on the fly
Yet my inner peace calms with ease

I am amused by sounds that are crude but true
I pleasure in things that are simple and clear
You laugh when I share things that I like about you
Yet it is my passion to be close to those who are dear

So when you measure your freedoms, measure them well
As the freedoms you have are not to be presumed
For the freedoms we have are too many to tell
I see them as gifts and blessings as well

If you don't believe me, walk in my shoes
And tell me what you see
You will be surprised to find as the freedoms you choose
Are determined by the restraints that cause you not to be free

By Eli Shaw

Inspired by Paul

This poem was inspired by Chapter 1, after reading and editing it so many times.

The Journey

When I was young,
I saw joy, possibilities and trust
As I got older
I began to see sadness, hate and disturbance in the dust

A young neighbor
Living with down syndrome
Became my friend
Because I found I needed to protect him

The neighbors' kids
Would taunt and tease him
Because he was different
And an easy target

I watched him
As he was pushed and shoved
And saw him smile
As he thought it was just a game of love

I took the blows
From the perpetrator's fist
And stood my ground
Until my friend moved away

That was a beginning
Of a journey I would come to know
To make right
What had been wronged and to let them know

I would stand up
To any injustice I see
If I say nothing
My actions they will see

The rest of my journey
I would record
In my mind and on paper
Which was my only sword.

By Eli Shaw

This poem was written many years ago when I was beginning to realize how big this AIDS thing was.

The Pandemic

Slowly the invading army draped its cloak
Layer by layer
Silently conquering the landscape like a plague
Without a prayer

The night leaves a layer of dust as the slumber keeps us warm
Only to awaken to find the invasion was successful
And the landscape gone

Wave after wave, they mutate as we trudge through the debris
Left by the invading army
Weighing us down day by day as we dig
Our way out anyway

Darkness looms over the fields with a moonlit glow To guide us
The romantic facade engulfs our imagination, hearts
And anticipation plus

Hope, shines her soft glow over the landscape
So barren
With her sounds and echoes reaching us with a beat
So random

It is then and only then our hearts and hopes
Are raised up
Knowing that everything we do will help to fill
The golden cup

Time comes and goes and yet stands still
As we heal together
Making strong our ability to fight this
Invisible lurking weather

Soon we will see a cure we say each day
With our dreams raising us high
And so we hold our values higher
So our dreams and hopes can fly

Our mission and passion are firm, to leave this place
A better place than we received it
As our children learn from our ways, mistakes and struggles
And learn where they will fit

It does not matter how we die or from what
As this invasion invisibly lurks
It is what we leave behind as tools for them to build
And work out all the quirks

Peace and calm is possible, but most always
Begins in the mind
And as our children nurture and care for this earth and all it is
She is already perfect as you will soon find

By Eli Shaw

This poem was inspired by the program I wrote called Legacy, and by listening to some of the students.

The Road to Legacy

As I have traveled this landscape of water, trees and sand
I have begun to reveal my SELF and its gears with
all its quirks and flaws to leave a trace

I have pondered the gift I have been given to reside in this place
And realize I have a choice which gives life so much grace

And a purpose we must find to love
Even if to us is not from above

My footprints, the legacy of the road and my feet
I choose the direction they point, to the fruits ahead so sweet

My choice, bathed in the juice of experience that has brought me this far
Laden with tears, fears and smiles and the occasional permanent scar

The path is long with stories to tell the children who grow,
The eyes of the small world around me are on
my every jolt and turn of my flow.

The images I will project on the corneas of their young mind,
Will last as my legacy will grow and shine.

What can I leave to those I leave behind as I choose my brand-new path,
Not can, but will, leave as I walk carefully and do the math.

Did I make a difference in the space I have moved?
As a sculpture does on the wood he has grooved.

Only if I ask will I know the truth that is within
As the blood flows under my skin

So remember the freedom of choice we have learned
from the legacy of frown or smile,
And to glow in the darkness as a light to lead
and turn that inch into a mile.

By Eli Shaw

This was written a few years after Mark died.

My Only Companion

The sound of a distant dog barking and the 4-second count of
Distant thunder,
My only companion

I had just received news of a friend's illness,
I decided to wander and let the cool night air heal me in its Stillness
My only companion

Many more have gone before, my well of tears all but dry,
As I sat on the bank overlooking the shore and waited for the Cry
My only companion

Three years have passed since that night took its toll,
Yet, though he be gone to another dimension,
I speak to him through my Soul.
My only companion

Eli Shaw

This poem was written after I spent time with Homer before I took him in as my son. I had only known him for a week.

Tell me Child!

Tell me child, what you're thinking
As the sun folds over the horizon

Your days are lifetimes as you fill
Each moment with the fresh smell of life

My days go quickly as I watch you unfold
Your world, and another day must end

Your journey, with your imagination as your guide
Takes you places I have long forgotten

Your play allows me a glimpse of the stardust and dreams
I once sprinkled on life

I, the person you look up to, and ask questions of,
Have traveled your journey

Only the scenery has changed
The trees have grown tall or disappeared

Tell me child, what you are thinking,
As the sun rises on your horizon

Our roads have met and another episode begins
Hold my hand, not tightly, as we walk a new path
In this garden of life

Tell me child…..

By Eli Shaw

This poem was written after finding out that one of my former students died by suicide. I worked with him in several situations. I knew his pain then, and yet saw him become strong and a vibrant soul. I remember thinking about how fragile he was with his situation and I knew he would have a long road. That road was cut short when his resolution to his pain became easier than the pain he was in.

Scott

Here I stand before you
A fragile creature among fragile creatures
Living on this fragile planet

Protected by the gravity that holds us
The air we breathe
Our superhero facades, beauty queen dreams
And egos

Our souls have cloaked us
With the protection
Of our silence
That we guard so carefully

Only to find
It calls us to our seclusion
And despair
As we breathe, some of the loneliest stand among us

Scotts time with us was short
But in that short time
He created a legacy of strength, love, compassion
And a gift so rare,
Himself

He was not a selfish person
He shared his knowledge
Love for nature
And his amazing spirit

He would never refuse to help others
Would offer it freely in fact
Encouraging others to do more than they thought they could
And give it his full attention

His life was short
But bright on the outside
Yet he found the strongest pain
To be life as we perceive it should be

It would only be Nature
With all its seasons that would be the quilt
That would caress this young man's soul
So perfect

His legacy will be short-lived
As we move through the twists and turns of our daily lives
Yet he leaves us a message, strong and loud
If we just stop to listen

The pains he endured
We may never grasp,
I assume are some of the same pains
We all share, protect and claim
As our own

We live our lives like little islands
In a sea of bubbles
Surrounding us in times of Turmoil
And afraid to touch

Not letting out the cries
Of our internal pain,
despair and helplessness
Is a defense and a fear
That no one will listen

We are not alone on this planet
By a long shot
Yet we stand as islands
Afraid to show our naked spirit

Scott, let us in many times
To his spirit dwelling
And still it was nature he could rely on
For most of his comfort

Yes, afraid to show the very essence of who we are

Why are we so afraid?

Where there is pain
There is also calm

Where there is despair
There is also joy

Where there is hate
There is also love

Where there is death
There is also life

Where there is hopelessness
There is also hope

Where there is me
There is also you

Where there is us
There is also them

Where there is helplessness
There is also help

Where there is nothing
There is also something

I stand here before you
My naked spirit
My soul open to ask the question
Why

I too do not like to expose my pain
As he didn't

Why?
The fear of being judged, pure and simple

Judge not

We all hide our secrets and pain
In a vault. in the deep reaches of our mind and soul
I know when MY vault is full
I feel the pain

I would only imagine
Scott's vault was full as I have known him since high school
And yet he was always fine
And put on a mask of calm

The natural world was his spiritual reality and solace
The human-made or fabricated things we hold
Are but the tools he used
To access that nature

I have also found
When I stuff my vault
There is always that one person
To help clean out my vault

Find that person in your life

I tend to clean my refrigerator
More often than my vault

I say to our friend Scott,
Brilliant and passionate
About so much
In life

You are not alone
You are loved
Your life is cherished

To those he left behind
Do not feel empty or lost with his absence
Scott has given us something
A gift
For each of us it is different
For each of us it is precious

Take time in your daily life to breathe
And smell nature
He will be right by your side
When you do

His mission is different now
His work is done here
The why's do not matter now
As you remember to....

Look for your pain
And find your calm

Look for your despair
And find your joy

Look for your hate
And find your love

Look for your mortality
And find your life

Look for your me
And find your you

Look for them
And find us

Look for your helplessness
And find your help

Look for your weakness
And find your strength

Do not let Scott's legacy fade lightly
He was not alone
Yet he was alone

We are not alone
Look and see who is with you.

Thank you, Scott,
For your legacy

Your good soul
Will be with me and those I meet
And may your pain be gone
And your calm eternal

By Eli Shaw

This poem was inspired by a friend of mine who asked me to write something creative for a poetry program, but the subject had to be about my collective experience with Alzheimer's.

Alzheimer's 101 In Eight Hours

4:00 PM   I come home and your bright familiar face shines with welcome home.

4:20 PM   I get dressed for dinner we are going to but cannot find my cufflinks. I call to you and you say they are with my cufflinks right in front of me. Silly me

4:40 PM   I call to you and ask you again what the address is we are going to once so familiar. You say, "It's your parents' house" and "I say oh yeah, I forgot."

5:00 PM   My keys don't seem to fit the car door and you tell me I am using the wrong one, once a task done unconsciously and not unfamiliar.

5:20 PM   I get mad at you for telling me I am driving in the wrong direction. You say, "Don't you remember where you grew up?" I am confused and let you drive.

5:40 PM   We get to my parent's house where I grew up. Much is familiar yet other things, unrecognizable like the swing I may have used. And when did they paint the house? You smile and usher me in.

6:00 PM   We are greeted by my father and a woman who says she
           is my step-mother who is unfamiliar to me. Dad says,
           "Here's mom." Thinking he is losing his mind I just agree
           with him.

6:20 PM   Suddenly two children appear, nephews I assume. I ask
           the one who looks more familiar who his friend is? He
           laughs and says "You are silly, Uncle Bob. I turn to the
           other but he is gone.

6:40 PM   We all sit at the table and I am surrounded by unfamiliar
           faces and unfamiliar food. The woman who claims to be
           my mom tells me it is my favorite dish. How would she
           know?

7:00 PM   Conversations seem muted and of a different language yet
           I know what they are saying. I tell myself to just agree and
           smile at everything.

7:20 PM   I see a picture on the wall of a guy who looks a bit like me
           but younger? I tell dad I do not know these people and he
           says, "It is you," and I say, "You must be mistaken."

7:40 PM   I am starting to find that just agreeing with everyone and
           saying yes, turns the noise down in my head. I see shadows
           but no people at times and figure it must be car lights.

8:00 PM   All of a sudden, I find myself in the living room where my
           friends would come over and we would watch TV together.
           I ask my dad, "Have you seen Jimmy?" he said, "Jimmy
           who?" I say, "Jimmy Smith." He says with a confused look,
           "He got married and moved to Germany." Then I look
           confused.

8:20 PM   I get mad and frustrated that he did not tell me. He is also too young to get married. Ten is definitely too young. I tell dad that he was just kidding with him.

8:40 PM   I am suddenly whisked away by people I don't know to a car. Tears are rolling down my face as I do not know where we are going. I say bye to the strangers and the car that smells, familiar but looks strange, drives off.

9:00 PM   We drive through a town I do not know and people wave to me from the sidewalk calling my name. The woman sitting next to me asks if I want to stop and pick up some whiskey, I laugh, as I am too young to drink.

9:20 PM   We drive on and come to a house with a number and a name. The name I think is mine but I do not know the number. Then the woman says, "We're home."

9:40 PM   I laugh and agree so I do not make them mad. I just keep smiling.

10:00 PM   She says, "Maybe you should get some sleep. You seem tired and confused. It is late also." I sit in the big comfortable chair and wait to see what she says again. She tells me to go upstairs and get ready for bed.

10:20 PM   I wander up the stairs and see several rooms. I pick one and sit on the bed. The woman comes in and takes my arm and guides me to a room much bigger. She mentions to me that I must be tired.

10:40 PM   She begins to undress. I look away. She helps me undress but I resist. I see she is crying.

11:00 PM   She tucks me in and she says goodnight as she slides under the covers on the other side of the bed.

11:20 PM   I feel bad because I do not know her. I think I should know her but my mind is so clouded. I close my eyes and suddenly everything is gone. My mind settles and calms me. I still see shadows.

11:40 PM   My mind wanders and I question, who this person is in me so many are concerned and crying about. Who are they? My world is in my mind, apart from the one they confuse me with. I am confused, and yet I am still the child I always was.

12:00 PM   As I sink into a slumber, caressed, only by pillows, I am gone.

Echoes of Others in My Past

I had worked with people with AIDS, cancer, and so many other illnesses for such a long time, and the loss of Mark led me into a world where I would meet some amazing individuals who had so much to say. I, as a photographer, had the idea to do a project called, If I Die Before I Wake, which would entail me photographing people who were infected with HIV and letting them tell their story. Many of them were willing to talk but not be photographed, as their physical appearance was quite different from when they were feeling well.

As I progressed with the project, I met many who eventually would not let me put what they said, in the exhibit, as it was too much to take in. They were afraid that some people they knew would see it and it would affect their friendships or relationships. HIV/AIDS was still not a very acceptable social issue, and there were many haters of people who were infected. The ones I was able to clear are in the following pages. The ones who signed off on the script and photo had died and his mother saw the exhibit and asked that her son's entry be taken down. Since then I have vowed to protect the living, even though the ones who have passed were willing to participate by using their first name and last initial only, and not to use their photos in any of the exhibits or books to follow, including this one.

What you will find are the first name and last initial of each participant and their script. It is sad that even to this day there is still a stigma, even when many celebrities have come forward. Unfortunately, it is the small guy who gets hurt. Thank you for understanding. Out of respect, I have given each their own page.

DAVID H.

Where do I go from here?

It's been a very tough fight, the last seven and a half years for me. I realize now that much pain and confusion has been enhanced by me. And me alone.

Where do I go from here? A lot of times I just don't know. I have learned through much pain and experience that the Almighty, works through other caring and spiritual people. This means that if I could do what's been so hard for me to do in the past, I could be better off than I am now.

The thing I must do is trust people more. Not trusting people comes from two things. One is the years I spend running the streets amid uncaring people. The other is the fear and looks an HIV-infected person gets when he/she takes a chance and speaks about being HIV-Positive. Being angry a lot of the time confuses me.

Where do I go from here? I often get stuck in being angry and waste much time, energy and then again get angry for allowing myself to get stuck again in the anger syndrome.

Through the seven and a half years I've been infected I've come to learn that a positive attitude is one of the best treatments to positively deal with being HIV. When my attitude isn't positive, I usually stay to myself. Sometimes isolation can become a problem. Especially when you're in a negative state of mind.

Today I still get lost and wonder, where do I go from here? I thank God for the people who care for another human being.

Because, others, along with my attitude, have brought me this far.

EVA J. "95"

I'm HIV Positive
I feel no sorrow and regret
Thank God I know
As I am knowing I am positive is a blessing

God loves me always
He knows my heart and goals
The love and understanding he shows me
Is indisputably blessed

I'm happy in my world of HIV
His expectation of all of us,
She or he, is to care for them
As a positive people in the world.

Mario and Patrick

The spring of our lives.

With every interaction in all our lives, we are left with an imprint, some good as well as bad.

The good we don't mind carrying around with us and the bad, well, it becomes very hard to get rid of. So, we carry it around as well.

When our lives touched, the weight of all our excess baggage that we brought to each other, weighed us down like an anchored ship, preventing us from growing and living. All we had was anger to express, and our gift to each other was blame.

The chain of our anger has finally been broken by the cold reality of HIV. We now share a love, a desire to live and yes, an illness. The seasons of our lives might now be short, but that's OK because we will "Live It" now.

Livingly, Mario and Patrick

DANA

Hi. My name is Dana. I am a Black female, 35, diagnosed with full-blown AIDS. T-cell count, 20. Two part-time jobs. Socially and physically active.

LIVING with the virus.

The way I live and see it is that without my faith in God, I could not be in the present physical and mental state of mind I am in. You know the saying that AA has: It won't work if you don't work it. Well, if you don't work, the Lord, He won't work you. I attend drop-in meetings. I also have all the things that a person with my medical status should have except for SSI which I turned down in order to maintain two part-time jobs.

What would I say to a person who has the virus? Don't let it get you. If you let it get you, you're gone. Quite frankly, I am enjoying life more so than I was before. I take time to notice things like looking at the trees on the street and the Hudson River. The New Jersey landscapes. I speak to my flowers more. I do a lot of things I normally took for granted.

What would I say my formula is for a good, healthy life? Take your medication, exercise, rest and thank God for each and every day you have here on this earth. Your attitude will definitely have to change. Things that normally aggravate someone, let them go. Who wants to die because your AT&T operator won't give you credit or you lose your credit cards? You can do this. If you can't, find someone who can or has, and listen.

LINDA

Linda is a person whose concern for others exceeds all boundaries of caring. With the loss in 1993 of her husband who was a strong force in the fight against AIDS, she has stepped out and spoken up.

Her fire can be sensed just by talking to her, but her love and concern outweigh all. When I asked what advice she would give to others, her answer was, "Get smart. Use a condom, damnit, and for God's sake, get tested!"

I asked her, "What was one of the hardest things you have encountered?" she said, "Telling my family through a letter was OK. Tough, but OK. Telling my mother tomorrow, in person, that's going to be tough."

I asked, "What do you hate the most about AIDS?" She said, "Having it."

DAVID D

David asked me to write for him, as his capacity to speak was greater than his ability to write. His attention span was usually not long. However, while I was talking to him, his remark to me was, "Keep talking while my brain is in gear." And it was in gear for over an hour.

When I told him the title of the show, he said, "I'll be happy if I wake before I die, and that goes for all of us. I hope we all wake up soon.

"My biggest upset in life, or regret, is that I allowed so many opportunities to slip by. That's why I'm doing this for the exhibit. I am not letting this one go by. I have wandered around aimlessly all my life and, on my way, I have wandered by so many people who have done and are doing so much good in life. It makes me feel small, and I do not like that. I feel like I have no voice anymore as I am HIV positive and who wants to talk to someone who is sick. I try to exist and sometimes it is so hard I ask myself why. Why do I want to exist? You have given me that answer, which is to tell my story, so others will not do what I have done or be like me. I was told one day that I am an inspiration and I could not understand how I could ever inspire anyone, but now I know. You have taught me so much about who I am in the Legacy Program and what I have to offer."

I asked him what he would like me to put into the script and he picked these few items as "it is limited space, and most of the other stuff is just existing crap and how I have failed in that respect. It is hard to talk to people with my mind wandering. They think I'm crazy. No, I'm just ill. Too bad they don't see that."

ROBERT M.

Robert asked me to write, as his facility with writing has become hampered lately.

His experience with losing friends has exhausted him. He loves life and the time he has here is for him but a weigh station on a journey with heaven as the destination.

In his words, "The destination is Heaven, yet we become troubled when the train begins to pull out." I said to him, "You're from the Old Guard." He replied, "Yes, when sex and our need for freedom and heroes were not yet diminished by the threat of AIDS. I spent much of my time at the hospital with those ready to pull out on the next train. My advice to anyone is to be honest with yourself and true to others. Our bodies are on loan to us. There is no early payment of the loan."

MARC H.

"Most people look at me kind of strange when I tell them that I thank God I'm HIV-Positive. But after living with HIV for nine years now, I know where my health and strength is coming from. HIV has given me a new life. I didn't see it before. I couldn't see it before, but I see it now. I believe that there are no coincidences in life, that everything has a purpose and things happen for a reason. I believe that we all have a part in God's master plan."

"For over 25 years of my life, I was suffering from alcohol and drug abuse. My life had no direction. I lived to use, and I used to live. No one told me that things could and would get better. I did not know how to deal with life on life's terms. I did not want to be responsible. I needed a wake-up call. God in his infinite mercy and grace did just that: He gave me a wake-up call.

I thank God today that I am now learning how to live according to his will. Through 12-step programs and other channels, I am able to enjoy all God's blessings. I don't think I would be where I am today had it not been for me being HIV-positive. So, I thank God for blessing me. And if I continue to live according to his will, I know that all will be well.

May God bless you as he's blessed me."

BONNIE

Our conversation was limited to small talk in the beginning, but gradually went into deeper subjects. I asked her about taking her picture, and if it would be all right. She agreed and seemed thrilled in her subtle way that I would want to. Knowing I was going to take the picture, she said she needed to paint her face. I could see where her face had weathered many storms in her life and now the biggest one, AIDS.

She said that her life wasn't a bed of roses and that it was full of pain at times, but her concerns were more about the people who didn't know about AIDS. She was affected by the same prejudices others have encountered, but hers were seen from a different angle.

Her experience prior to getting admitted to the nursing home was a near-death experience. She said, "I got so close to the end. I began to see things differently and wished I had done some things differently." She spoke a little about her 9-year-old daughter and her concern for her, but I could see it was a hard subject for her to talk about. Her pain was evident.

I asked her finally, "What is the one thing that bothers you the most about AIDS and all of its facets?" She hesitated a bit, and after a struggle with her eye shadow, she said, "You know, those people who are afraid of me using the bathroom because of me being HIV-positive. They don't understand. How do they think I feel? I should be the one with the fear. I am the one that can catch anything at any time and die from it. I get so afraid of the fact that I could contract even the smallest virus or germ and they look at me like I was dirt. They don't understand. They don't understand at all."

This next one was in response to a questionnaire I sent out to the AIDS community. He sent this to me and agreed to meet with me for coffee later. He turned out to be an amazing human being with such a great presence.

TOMMY

1. How do you feel about someone asking questions about something as personal as an illness, in this case, AIDS or cancer?
A. It depends on who the person is.

2. How long have you been positive?
A. 4 years.

3. What were your thoughts when you were told?
A. Shocked.

4. What were your greatest fears before you became HIV-positive?
A. Jobs, money, jail.

5. What is your greatest fear now?
A. Dying.

6. What was your outlook on life before?
A. Bright.

7. What is it now?
A. Gloomy.

8. Are you angry?
A. Yes

9. Do you get angry often?
A. I keep it under control with medicine – it's always inside me though.

10. Do you know what makes you angry?
A. Yes, people who are full of bullshit.

11. What does your anger make you feel like?
A. It makes me want to hurt people. But I don't.

12. At whom or what do you direct your anger?
A. I don't direct it. I medicate it

13. Do you feel better?
A. Yes, when I am medicated.

14. Do you have the courage and where do you think it comes from?
A. Yes, God.

15. Outside of what everyone tells you, how long do you think you have?
A. Less than two years.

16. Have you expressed this to your loved ones?
A. Yes

17. Do you find forgiveness easy or hard?
A. Hard

18. Do you still have dreams and ambitions? If so what are they?
A. Yes. To have my VA pension reinstated and good safe sex.

19. What do you think about death?
A. I'm afraid.

20. Have you planned for it and what would you like it to be like?
A. I haven't planned too much. I want to die with little or no pain.

21. In your final hours who would you like to be at your side?
A. Only my family.

22. Who are you?
A. Just a 39-year-old white guy.

23. What is your fondest memory?
A. My girlfriend. She's dead.

24. What would you like to say to those you love?
A. Thanks.

25. To the world?
A. You suck! The way you treat people who have AIDS or are different, Sucks.

26. What are your feelings about the progress of AIDS research?
A. Research Progress? Bullshit. It's all about money and what part of society you are living in.

27. What do you think about the ignorance concerning AIDS?
A. Not much. That's the way of the world.

JANET

My fondest memories were of spending time with my family back when I was 10 to 15 years old. I remember the fun I had playing with my cousins and my sister when we used to talk about things in the past, or play house or football.

We were a close family. I remember I was very loved and respected by my cousins and they looked to me for advice and to settle arguments. I felt loved even though I was adopted. They never treated me different. I remember the fun my sister, and I had when we played and competed for boys as teenagers. Although sometimes we hurt each other, I thought of imagining not having a sister to yell at, fight with, and disagree with, and how that would be different.

It would be difficult to hug her and put my arms around her or to be able to feel her arms around me and know that she will always be there for me no matter what life has to offer me. That she can accept me being HIV-Positive and still be my sister above all, means a lot to me. She has been my hard rock. She knows that life for me has not been easy. She knows that I wasn't a bad person and I know it hurts her to know that one day I may not be here and that she would have no one to share her hurt with like her sister.

I would like for her to forgive me for lying about the house we were going to have together with our kids and I would like to confess to her that I didn't mean to hurt her by having this virus and for leaving her before we were able to get our house together. You are my best friend. You are the greatest in my eyes and will always be.

I love you Maria. To my girls, remember that just because Mommy is HIV-Positive, it doesn't mean that she was bad but that life is important and never take advantage and always respect that Mommy loves you always and forever. To my Mom and Dad, thank you for loving me when no one else did.

DENIS S

When Denis responded to my questions, they came from a questionnaire I sent out to see what I would get back. Many of these questions were hard to come up with and ask. As I was told, they were just as hard to answer. I felt they were important, and many of them came from people who were HIV-Positive and told me that these were the questions that they would rather be asked and answer, instead of the looks and stares that dominated the social atmosphere of people with the virus. This is what I got back from Denis, who by the way is such an amazing person and had a lot to say in some of the writings I had read that he had written.

1. How do you feel about someone asking questions about something as personal as an illness, in this case, AIDS or Cancer?

A. I have no problem with it. I want to talk about it and even try to obliterate the stigma of it while I am able.

2. How long have you been diagnosed?

A. Since 1994 with my first T-cell count (officially).

3. What were your thoughts when you were told?

A. I wasn't ill at the time, so it was a bit easier to, but with what was to happen to me, I was unsure.

4. Do you have a family that supports you?

A. Yes, luckily, they are not AIDS-phobic.

5. How long did it take for them to accept the fact that you were HIV-Positive?

A. None of us had that much of a chance, I was in a wheelchair from neuropathy and lymphoma of the liver within a matter of three months.

6. What were their questions and fears?

A. A lot of medical questions as we went along, always keeping the faith.

7. When did you feel comfortable telling others or have you yet?

A. I've always wanted to talk about my life, my experiences and interact about my illness.

8. In general, what is the usual reaction after telling someone?

A. I try to gently reflect, like in a mirror, that my time is valuable and precious, I am fighting but I'm probably going to die sooner or later.

9. What were your greatest fears before you became HIV-Positive?

A. That I wouldn't be recognized for my work, (my art), at all, before I died.

10. What is your greatest fear now?

A. The same, but I'm really working on it as much as possible.

11. What was your outlook on life before?

A. Hedonistic but loving. I gave my longtime lover passage from this life as well. He passed on May 2nd, 1995.

12. What is it now?

A. Still to try to create and be recognized, Produced and appreciated.

13. Are you angry?

A. Yes, very much so.

14. Do you get angry often?

A. It depends on the person, thought, situation or memory.

15. Do you know what makes you angry?
A. Homophobia, "AIDS phobia", ignorance, greed and cruelty.

16. What does your anger feel like?
A. It bristles. My anger, my violence is bristling.

17. At who or what do you direct your anger?
A. Unfortunately, often at the ones I love the most.

18. Do you feel better after your anger is gone?
A. Yes, I've learned through it hopefully.

19. Where do you think courage comes from and do you have it?
A. I'm told I have a lot of courage, I never would have known.

20. Outside of what everyone tells you, how long do you think you have?
A. God, I keep praying and hope till age 40. I am 35 now.

21. Have you expressed this to your loved ones?
A. Yes. In a number of ways. I haven't planned a funeral.

22. Do you find forgiveness easy or hard?
A. It depends again, on the person, or situation actually.

23. What do you plan to do with the rest of your life?
A. Expose the "real heathens," create and laugh with friends and try to create more "art."

24. Who is your greatest support?
A. My mother and a few special, close friends along with some medical people.

25. Have you told them they are your greatest support?

A. I think they know. I about died on Sept 10, 1994. I had an infinite amount of support from my lover, family, and friends.

26. Do you still have dreams and ambitions?

A. Yes, I will not let anyone or anything make me lose my dreams.

27. What are your dreams and ambitions?

A. To be heard, seen and appreciated for my work which is in a transition phase.

28. How do you feel about these questions at this point?

A. They're just fine. I am enjoying this.

29. What do you think about death?

A. I hope I'll make it welcome and it'll make it easy for me to do that passage or transition.

30. Have you planned for it and what would you like it to be like?

A. I just want to go to sleep to be perfectly honest.

31. In your final hours who would you like to be at your side?

A. A man really!! My lover was with his father.

32. It has been said that people who are quite ill have been able to find their inner selves. Have you?

A. Yes, maybe not quite enough yet though.

33. Where do you come from?

A. Born in N.J. then grew up in N.Y. State and returned from my teen years on.

34. What is your fondest memory?
A. Being complimented on my first film I made as a kid.

35. What would you like to say to those you love, those you don't love and the world in general? Be as profound as you wish.
A. When all else fails, laugh!! Be kind and true to yourself always.

36. What are your feelings about the progress of AIDS research?
A. It's so hard to tell, with all of its revenue, all the lies.

37. If you didn't have AIDS what do you think you would be doing?
A. Trying to create more art and writing.

38. Do you think positive more than negative?
A. I've always retained a "gothic" outlook on life.

39. If someone wrote a plaque to honor your greatest deed, what would it say?
A. "As kind as they get."

40. What was the highest point of your life so far?
A. Falling in love for the first time.

41. There have been many instances where people have tried or succeeded in committing suicide. What would you say to them?
A. Think it out completely.

42. What were your thoughts about AIDS before you became positive?
A. My friends have about all died, on and around me, for 11 years. I knew we were in a plague.

43. If you met someone who just became positive, what would you say to them and would you give them any advice?

A. It can get better. Relax and prepare for many things, good and bad.

44. Let's say that today was going to be a totally positive day, what would it be like?

A. "Finishing" creative projects.

45. Some people have left videos for their loved ones. Is it a good idea and if you did this, what would you say to them?

A. I love you and remember me as a good thing.

46. What do you think about the ignorance concerning AIDS?

A. It may never end, I pray it does though. It'll help a lot of children.

47. Do you have any questions?

A. No. Thank you for your time! God bless you for your work and love!!

Signed,
Warmly
Denis S

THE LOST MANUSCRIPTS

Just as a note before you read this essay. I wrote this in 1994. It was my first attempt at writing this book and was not long after I lost Dad and Mark. I wanted someone to edit it or give me some feedback, so I sent a copy of the whole manuscript to my sister. July 2, 2018, my sister found it again in a box. To me, this was like the dead sea scrolls, as amongst my many moves, this and several other chapters were lost. Stolen computers did not help any. That is why I copy everything many times now. I read it and realized I have included some of the content in some recent essays, as I did not think I would ever see them again. Talk about fate. Here it is. Twenty-four years later. Thanks, Nancy, I will never judge anyone who holds onto stuff again.

THE TRAINING OR,
WHO ARE THE CAREGIVERS?

In February 1992, I had received a call from my sister, Nancy. She had been staying in Florida with my father, who had been undergoing many tests to find out what was wrong with him. He had been quite congested from several things, and was going through anxiety attacks one after the other. The call was full of good news. She told me that my father was coming home to undergo an operation to get a new valve, "a valve job" as we commonly referred to it later.

There were many people involved in the caregiving process concerning Dad, such as nurses, doctors, and family. But there were many we didn't acknowledge as Caregivers. Many of the distant family members and family friends were now considered Caregivers, as well as neighbors we hadn't seen in that caregiving position. Yet they were all also Caregivers in one way or another. Talking to many of the people who knew my father, I got the feeling they were also sort of Caregivers, even though they were not directly involved with him or the family. What I was finding out, and now understand deeply, was that just by calling my father and wishing him well, they were Caregivers also. They wouldn't have the same emotion as the family or close friends, but after his death, they too had a deep sense of caring and loss just from the kind words and flowers they were able to give him. My father was what they called a prognosticator, which means he would predict the weather and they would put his predictions in the paper along with another resident. They were in competition so to speak, and each season for a couple of weeks the boxing gloves were on, and because of this and his visibility and kind works in the community, many people felt they knew him well. He never refused to respond to a friendly "Hi" or, "How's the weather, Bob?"

I knew I had to get my things together and make sure someone would be there if Mark needed anything. Mark was in his advanced stages of AIDS. I got my things and packed the car. I knew it was going to be a rough ride, not only from the anxiety and both needing help, but there was a huge snowstorm on the way. I left the house figuring it would only be a 3-hour drive. Then the snow hit about 20 minutes into the drive. It was about to be a hell of a ride. After driving 6 ½ hours in the snow to be with my father before he went into the hospital, I began a journey which many had taken before me and many more would take after me. When I arrived at my father's house, he was in the kitchen sorting through papers and items on the table. I sat with him as we talked for a while and exchanged thoughts we had never shared before. His concern for Mark having AIDS was deep, which I now saw clearly, and I also began to see him as Mark's Caregiver too. His words and support, even knowing he was going to be operated on the next day and knowing it would be risky, were things I have carried with me since that day and they also would be an indirect aid to my caring for Mark.

He and Mark had spoken many times on the phone and were co-supportive in so many ways. Unfortunately, I was a major concern to both of them, which I did not know until later. If I had known then, I think I would have been upset, as "I was the Caregiver, not the victim." Since then I have found that being a Caregiver also includes being a victim of sorts. I have heard it said that when one is sick, there are usually many more who will need help. There is a lot of truth in this phrase.

It was getting late, and we had to get up early as he had some stops to make before he got to the hospital. I remember my father in the living room, which had been converted into a bedroom. Nancy and I had spent many hours working out the wrinkles of how it would have to be comfortable and easy for the nurses to come in and work with Dad. The silence in the house which I grew up in was deafening. There were some sounds like the clicks of the heaters, as if someone was tapping on them, the tick-tock of the many clocks he had, and a myriad of small noises like the wind, and snow hitting the windows, that caused a symphony of memories to seep through the cracks and corners of the room I desperately tried to sleep in.

My father also grew up in this house and had previously been sorting out many photos and items of his youth which he was eager and willing to show to anyone. Dad is on the West Warwick Historical Society, or as he sometimes referred to as the Hysterical Society, as they all had such a great time together and loved keeping old things, as I do now. Not being able to fall asleep, I sat up and began to look through some of the things which were so much a part of his life and his soul. The background music had now become the irregular snores of my father, which he was famous for.

For the first time, I began to understand a lot about who my father was. He was not just my father, but now was also my friend and a wonderful, compassionate, and kind human being who was so full of love, life, and caring. I began to see where I got many of my traits and habits, especially the art of collecting. That is another story. I saw a bit of my mother in him, who had died 10 years earlier. How he coped with so many things in his life was remarkable to me. We seldom understand this until we go through the loss of someone we have connected with for some time. This I would see even more clearly after Mark's death.

I think of my father as a silent teacher. He had a way of teaching things with his soft-spoken manner and voice which I still remember as he sat at the top of the stairs with sis and me. He would read to us at night when we were very young. I also remember his work with youth, especially in Cub Scouts where he was well respected for his compassion, soft-spoken and caring personality. So many young scouts would go on to remember him in many ways, but mostly as a mentor. He was one of the few scoutmasters at that time who received the Beaver Award, which is one of the highest awards you can get in scouting. Those thoughts rushed through my head as if making room for more as quickly as possible. Photographs on the table revealed a man I didn't know, yet knew profoundly. I began to see how I had taken so much of my father's love for granted. A little bit of guilt began to filter in, but not for long, as there were so many pictures. The legacy he would leave when he died was enormous, yet as with my mother who commanded overtime during her wake as there were so many people coming to see her, the legacy would die out with the people she, and he affected when they grew older. I am sure we all would want to be remembered with a long-lasting Mister Clean legacy, but unless something tangible is left to recall who you were, like ink in water, it will fade and dilute into the fabric of life.

That night went by slowly. I was able to see the sun come up and share what was to be my last morning talk with my father. His hopes and dreams were spilling out of his mouth, knowing that this operation would give him a little more time to get his life in order and make a difference, even more than he had done already. The sun burst into the kitchen on the table where we shared coffee and cereal, and a sense of unity I had not experienced with him before. I didn't understand why, but I went on autopilot as if nothing else in the world mattered except that moment. I still carry that feeling with me when I can, as it helped me when I was helping Mark as well as myself making each moment count.

Dad was ready to go, but we had to visit my brother in Cranston before we got to the hospital. I was seeing that my father had to do as many things as he could, cramming for the final so to speak before he had the operation, just in case there was a problem. This was another thing I didn't understand, but am fully aware of now. That meeting with my brother Don was so intense and important to all of us, and I wouldn't see why until Dad's death.

After leaving Don, we were on our way. I noticed he was sort of meditating. He asked me to not speak for a while. He later told me he had learned to ease his anxiety by closing his eyes and thinking of cool, calm, thoughts while breathing slowly. Like I said before, he was a silent teacher. I later began to use this method to help me through Mark's ordeal, as well as many others.

I met my sister at the hospital, and we admitted my father. When he was settled in, my sister and I went to the house to finish setting up the living room to our Dad's needs. What we didn't know was that he would never return. The next day he was operated on. The operation was a success, which pleased us all.

Later that day we got a call from the hospital. My father had coughed up his breathing tube and slipped into a coma. A coma was a new experience for me, and was the beginning of what was to be a long period of going on autopilot again. We all seemed to just be concerned with immediate needs and doing what was important at the time and nothing else. I was in constant contact with Mark. He was quite concerned with my mental state at the time. He would talk me down to a calmer level at times which gave me a new boost to go on with what was happening and deal with the pain and emotional distress I was not addressing. I am sure he could see through my words each time we spoke. I also did not know at the time that he was slowly getting worse. Even though he was working 60 hours a week, it was painful, and he was beginning to swell in some areas of his body. He would just tell me not to worry and to deal with my father.

Dad was in a coma for quite a while, and each day we could see him slowly get worse. The operation was so successful that his heart had never been stronger. His brain was not functioning, and he needed total support. We began talking to him and telling him all the things that were happening in the family and the world. Of course, there were funny things that happened which saved our sanity, but we were still on autopilot and holding on as best as we could.

I went to the house one day and picked some flowers from his garden. He was one of the best gardeners I will ever know. When I got back to the hospital, I placed them in my father's hand and rubbed them on his fingers and palms. I put them up to his nose, hoping he could smell them. I noticed his face twitched a bit which made me think he could smell them. The doctor told me later that it was just an involuntary reaction. I placed them on the table next to his bed with a few other items I had found in and around the house. One was a stone my nephew found in the driveway, something of my mother's, some pictures, and his coffee cup that still had dried coffee in it. I knew inside that this was more for me than him, as he could not see them as far as I knew. Looking back, I think how trivial all those gestures were, but it helped.

The support of the nurses was unbelievable. I knew it was their job, but I could see a little of themselves come through their starched white uniforms. They were real troopers and told us we were as well.

I was sitting at the foot of the bed reading one morning. The sun had come out and was unusually bright for that time of year, and especially after the storm which had left the air crisp and clear. I am sure I could have read into that experience pretty far, but I just felt the warmth of the sun at that time. The radio next to my father's head facing his good ear as he called it, was playing a song I knew my mom loved. The unit was quiet, and no one was around except one nurse. Looking up at my father's face I noticed him crinkle his nose, which he did periodically. The nurse said it was a normal muscle reflex reaction as there was still living in his brain stem. His eyes were open and moving a bit. I sat up and held his hand. The swelling in his face and arms made him look like Popeye or Ed Asner. That song, the nose twitch, and his eyes sent my imagination on a roller coaster ride of emotions. For the first time in some weeks, I felt he connected on some level.

Then without warning, his eyes teared. For that moment there was just him, mom and me in the world. Nothing else mattered. The nurse saw this and knew it might have upset me. She checked his vitals and a few things as I said he was starting to look like Popeye. She said," I should bring in a pipe tomorrow." That broke the ice and made me laugh. She was a regular nurse, and we had gotten to know each other well. That brought me back down to earth. She knew I would joke around some, so the joke was ok.

The days and nights went by slowly. I had been sleeping in the recliner chair most nights. Many questions had to be answered and decisions made. Those were the toughest days when we had to make decisions about him off life support, raising questions like, "What happens when we do?" My sister and brothers and I were closer than we had ever been. It seemed that good comes out of tragedy sometimes, and we were learning the hard way.

The day came when we had to decide when to take him off the respirator. Not knowing what the outcome would be, we consulted with the doctor. After the decision was made, we felt it was important that the grandchildren see him first. That was a rough one to go through, as he and mom practically raised them at times. They were extremely close. Would it affect them negatively, or would they be able to handle it? We decided it was time, and called them in. Before they saw him, we briefed them with one of the nurses as to what they would see, and that it might be the last time they would see him alive, if that is what one could call his state of being.

They were as ready as they would ever be. They slowly came in, quiet and scared. Donny walked right up to the bed and held his grandfather's hand, not talking and just barely breathing. We let him know that it was ok to touch him and talk to him, as he might be able to hear him. Kristi stood at the foot of the bed with her arms around me tight and secure. I took her over to the machines and talked about what they did. Donny was fascinated with the graph on the screen showing his heartbeat. He called it the TV.

After a few minutes, which seemed like an eternity, we let them say whatever they wanted to say to Grandpa, as it would possibly be their last chance. Tears were shed, and we walked them back to the waiting room where we talked about it. One of the nurses came in and helped us with the dialogue. I couldn't imagine what was going on in their young minds. I knew it would be an experience that would make them stronger. I didn't envy them. Yet what they were able to do was more than most would ever have the opportunity to do in a lifetime. To have the chance to be complete with the person most meaningful in their young lives was special.

What they were about to lose was more than I could imagine. This was the person who helped teach them good from bad, showed them things no one else could, shared things and experiences only grandfathers can and gave them a start in life only he could give. But most of all, this was the person who showed them the meaning of unconditional love that would hopefully last throughout their lives. I am proud to say, it has.

The time came when we had to turn off the respirator. My sister, brother and I held each other with our cousin Joan's assistance. She was a nurse and had helped Dad more than anyone could have and more than we could ever know. Her experience as a nurse and ICU worker was invaluable. We stood and waited. The light went on, the machine went off, and we glued our eyes to the screen to see what would happen. A few seconds went by without a breath, and then it happened. He began breathing on his own. Go figure.

My sister Nancy and I took shifts while my brother Tom went to get his children, who were quite young then. We didn't know what to do or where to go, so we just sat and waited. I felt like I was on a death watch. I was. While I was sitting there, I thought about the day my mother had a stroke and a heart attack. I was working in Massachusetts when I got the call. I was a house attendant for a group home for mentally challenged people. One of my coworkers was a psychologist and helped me tremendously. He had a teaching manner much like my dad's, calm and nurturing. I did not get the chance to be complete with my mom, so I was damn sure I was going to be complete with dad. I even shared what I wanted to tell her with him the night before the operation. It was like he could take that information and tell her if the operation did not go well.

Suddenly, the beeps were getting erratic, and his eyes opened as he gasped for air. I felt helpless. My sister dropped the book she was reading, and we just sat there gasping with him as if we would be able to assist him in that way. We looked at each other, helplessly waiting for the last breath. His eyes looked like they knew we were there and we both tried to talk to calm him and ourselves and make the transition as comfortable as possible.

I have never had so many emotions going on at one time. I felt like I was going with him. I didn't want him to go, but I didn't want him to continue as he was. We both had to let go at that point. The beep went to a single hum, and his breathing slowly subsided. Then as if coming up for air, he gave one last gasp and went limp.

I didn't know it then, but what I had just gone through was almost a training course for me, as I would soon have to go through a similar event in a few months. As I look back at it all, I see how experiences in our lives prepare us for all the stuff we must attend to later. I had no idea how important all this and the events to follow like the funeral, meeting family and friends, etc. would be in my ordeal with Mark's illness and ultimate death.

I felt like I was going through a reality check all the while on autopilot. I had to learn to set priorities as they came to the top of the list and deal with them one by one. As I said before, it sometimes takes a tragedy to allow the good in life to show its face.

I guess there are hundreds of sayings or wise thoughts I could paraphrase at this point. But I think I would like to leave that up to you. During that time of taking care of Dad and Mark, going through their things, meeting people I never knew who knew me from the stories he told them about his children or they knew us when we were small, finding out that they had so many people who could be considered Caregivers at some point, and looking at all the people in my life who have at one time or another done a good deed for me or helped me with an issue, I started to realize that we are all Caregivers in some way. Who are the Caregivers? Look around you and see who has helped you get to this point in your life, not just parents or grandparents, but ancestors, siblings, neighbors, friends, and yes sometimes enemies, teachers, nurses, doctors, bus drivers, politicians, priests and ministers, parish people, and on and on. Anyone who has at one time paid you a compliment which made you feel good so you did better, or gave you a discount when you did not have enough change, or recognized you for some good work you did in the community, or made you feel good when you were down, or told you something you did not want to hear but needed to hear to get to the truth, and I could go on. All these people are Caregivers of sorts. And then there are the ones like myself who get paid for it, or take care of a family member as an obligation no matter how little financial, medical, or emotional support they get. These are the unspoken heroes to so many people I have spoken to. They usually say "I do not know what I would have done without them." Yet we do not tell them that. In most cases, the pay that a PCA will receive is on the low end, and they usually do not rack up 40 hours a week, yet they are there, day in and day out.

I guess what I am saying is that we need to recognize as many of the people in our lives who are willingly giving of themselves and say thank you. Hey, that makes you a Caregiver too.

SUPPORT?

When Mark was ill, there were many times I thought, "I wish I had some support." At that time I didn't know what support looked like. I thought support was having a professional, a doctor, a psychologist, or someone with some degree who could give me some technical feedback. What I wasn't aware of was that I had a wealth of support from family, friends, and just watching TV. Also, I didn't realize that Mark was my greatest support.

There are those of you who have gone through more horrifying experiences in life and can say I was lucky. This I know, and I am not trying to compare battle scars. What I believe I am trying to do is to convey the fact that no matter how tough things get, and no matter how alone we feel, there is always support out there. Even during the death camps in WWII or the slave ships where there was no foreseeable support, there was still hope. Sometimes we must ask for it, and other times it just happens, but always, hope is there. Hope and support also have many faces and depending on how open you might be to them, will make the difference as to how you receive support or embrace the hope.

I was on the caregiving end of things, and I am sure that Mark felt like support was non-existent at times also. But looking back at it all, I have become aware of support as being everywhere I look. I must make that step to attain it, and as long as I can see it as support, it works.

Being on what I have called autopilot sometimes places blinders on our vision of who and what support is. It also inhibits asking for help. It might be shame or embarrassment or ego which keeps us from saying, "Could you help me with something?" When I began to look around and remove the blinders, I began to see how much support there was out there. I would have given my right arm for a list or guide book to go by. Unfortunately, the rules of the game change every day, and this made me feel like I was the only one in the room.

We have to want to be helped to get it, and I guess I was in the "I don't need it" phase of the experience many times. I believe it is called denial. I also thought that everyone must know what I was going through and couldn't understand why they didn't offer their help. It is hard to ask, and at times I didn't.

It wasn't until the day we had to take him to the hospital that I felt I needed to ask. Mark's skin was turning yellow, and he called me into the room. He asked me to open the blinds, as it was making him look yellow. When I opened the blinds, I noticed he was indeed yellow, and a sense of fear I have never known came over me. Helpless and scared, I called the doctor and told him what was happening.

The doctor was furious that I hadn't called earlier and ordered me to get him to the hospital. Mark was having a hard time breathing, and the fear was intense. I called an ambulance to see if they would transport him to the hospital, which was in the next town. They couldn't go into the other town, for some rule or regulation had prohibited it. I then called the hospital, and they said I would have to call the EMS in my town. I then called the EMS back and pleaded with them, but it wasn't going to happen.

I then asked if they would send two guys over to help get him into the station wagon so I could get him into the hospital. They agreed to do that. When they got to the house, I could see the shock on their faces when they met him. He was swollen and yellow. But they put all that aside and got him into the car while Mark was screaming with pain. If it wasn't for their help, I don't know what would have happened. I only wish I knew who they were so I could thank them personally instead of calling the EMS and thanking them in general, which I did.

When we arrived at the hospital, he was rolled into a room where the doctor worked with him. I was so proud of Mark for his courage. I know a lot of it was for me. They realized the cavity around the lungs was filling with fluid, which was why he couldn't breathe. They told him they were going to drain it and asked me to hold him. Some of the staff knew him from a previous visit and were stunned at his condition.

I leaned over and he put his arms around my shoulders. Then they put a long needle in, and he began to drain. I could see that the struggle Mark was going through, and my curiosity overcame my sense of nausea. They took over three quarts of fluid out of him. Someone made a joke about a filling station and said, "Fill her up with high test." With that, the atmosphere in the room lightened up.

Joking around seemed to be a way of handling it all as we all sort of knew that he may not be going home again. When they finished, they kept him there for more than a few hours. I can only guess why. There seemed to be an issue as to where he was to go from here.

I had an exhibition going on that night, and it was the opening. It was something Mark was excited about. He told me that I should go and get ready for the opening, as I needed to get changed and be there early. He felt so bad that it was also the day he was admitted to the hospital. I went up to the room he would be in for the rest of his life, to get him settled. He was put into the hospice section where it was like a real bedroom. I kept stalling, as I didn't want to leave him, but he finally kicked me out.

The ride home seemed longer than it should have. A part of me was missing, but I had to get my act together as the exhibit opening was in an hour or so. I was so busy thinking of what was happening to Mark, but I made it on time. This was a show that Mark wanted to see. I had to take pictures so he would not miss them.

I got to the show and got settled. I had sent out over 400 invitations that month and was not sure if many would come because it was in July when a lot of people were on vacation. No more than ten people came, but they were good friends, and it was good to be with people who cared about me. They had heard about Mark, and they knew it was hard, so they got me drunk on the wine I had ordered. Three of my favorite girls from the church were there - Nellie, Janet, and Julie who were my biggest support in so many ways. They would do little things for me that would make life a little easier to handle. Brownies on my doorstep, lunch, a bottle of wine, and just some good conversations were just what the doctor ordered.

The night was long, and I stayed until it was over. I went back to the hospital where I sat with Mark until the early morning hours. Sleep was just another word at this point. I knew I was going to spend a lot of time there and asked Mark what he needed me to bring him for the stay there. Of course, he had a list ready, and it was up to me to find everything. The list consisted of books, some files, medication, pictures, and a host of other items which meant a lot to him. I began to realize that my job was now to make him as happy and comfortable as possible. Nothing else mattered. In the weeks to come, he would have tests and meetings with doctors and a final goodbye meeting with his friends and family. That was the most important thing to him, completing the time he had with friends and family.

The rest of this chapter has been covered, where he died in the hospital. I want to emphasize that no matter how troubled you are or difficult your caregiving experience is, if you look for support you can find it. The key is that you have to be ready to receive it.

THE FUTURE
OF THE CAREGIVING WORLD

One of my concerns about the future of caregiving is that because of the growing older population and the younger population declining in numbers, the reliance of family and friends to stand in as caregivers is increasing. When people were not living as long, there was less chance that they would show signs of dementia and Alzheimer's and other illnesses that develop later in life. Now, with the extended life span, the population of people needing care is growing. The attitude towards the caregiving population, concerning wage issues is becoming more and more prevalent. Many of the situations where it is a family member who has taken on the role of caregiver, leaving a job or sacrificing their lifestyle to make sure their elder is comfortable, has increased also because of lack of insurance and finances to use a facility or hire home care programs. This can cause many issues as the people involved are too close to the individual being cared for and can lead to very uncomfortable moments including anger and frustration.

In 2015 the Family Caregiver Alliance estimated that there were 43.5 million caregivers who have provided unpaid care to an adult or child. That estimate is growing in leaps and bounds. Unfortunately, with the uncertainty of the political atmosphere in health care, I do not see anything changing very quickly.

If it were not for the volunteer workers, we would be in a lot of poop. They are the heroes in my mind. It is going to take a lot of bipartisan work and public support to make it all work. One of the main reasons I wrote this book was to shed light on the extent of the caregiving world and how it can be applied to all facets of life. We are all caregivers in some way at some time in our lives.

Some of the organizations who make life a bit easier and help with collecting information and training are the Family Caregivers Alliance, Administration on Aging and the US Department of Veterans Affairs. These vital support vehicles are here to be used by everyone.

So for now, as we lunge forward into the future realm of caring with all its curves and straightaways, we must pool all our resources and communicate as I have done with this book, about our experiences, highs and lows so that others who are just coming on the scene can have a head start.

Lyrics to the song Memories

From the Broadway Musical Cats

Midnight not a sound from the pavement
Has the moon lost her memory?
She is smiling alone
In the lamplight, the withered leaves collect at my feet
And the wind begins to moan

Memory, all alone in the moonlight
I can smile at the old days
I was beautiful then
I remember the time I knew what happiness was
Let the memory live again

Every streetlamp seems to beat
A fatalistic warning
Someone mutters and the street lamp gutters
And soon
It will be morning

Daylight
I must wait for the sunrise
I must think of a new life
And I mustn't give in.

When the dawn comes
Tonight will be a memory too
And a new day will begin

Burnt out ends of smoky days
The stale cold smell of morning
A streetlamp dies; another night is over
Another day is dawning

Touch me!
It's so easy to leave me
All alone with my memory
Of my days in the sun

If you touch me,
you'll understand what happiness is
Look, a new day has begun.

Andrew Lloyd Webber

These are the lyrics of the song, Memories from the Broadway musical Cats. After reading them, I could not understand why Mark wanted to use that song in the hospital to share with us. There are so many hopeful phrases that celebrated days to come as well as the memories. He knew he only had a few weeks or days left. When I revisited the video of Elaine Paige's performance of the song as Grizabella, an old, tattered grumpy creature who few wanted to entertain as a friend or acquaintance and even though the others seemed to mock her almost to the end, I began to see something different.

In the song she sings of how all she has left are her memories of days gone by and the quiet and lonely streets where the street lamps are the time keeper to when the morning will begin. She seems to cry out to others to see her as not just a creature but a part of their community. She begs them to touch her as it is easy to see her and if they do, she could show them want happiness is as she has experienced so much of it. But now she is old and this is all anyone is willing to see.

As she reluctantly realizes another day has begun, a moment that should bring joy and promise only evokes fear and pain for her in her last days.

Suddenly one of the other cats comes over and dares to touch her which immediately creates a sense of admiration and compassion between the two. She becomes real to the other cats. She is now looked at as a soul with a legacy to leave. She is respected for going trough what they will inevitably someday go through and kindly send her off to that somewhere we all imagine differently.

I now realize what I saw in Marks eyes and voice when he died. I was too busy with my ego and counting my losses emotionally and physically to experience him at that moment. It was not until the last hours of his life that we truly shared what he was feeling and I was able to receive what he was sharing. It was like he was saying that there is not much time left so let's make the best of it and just put your ego elsewhere.

This is so visible in our interactions with the homeless citizens in our towns and cities. How many times have you passed by a homeless person and looked the other way? I can't count the times when I was guilty of this act. I did change that and began to say at least hi to them. Then I started to talk to them and eventually I would bring something for them to eat. I have to say that it is a process and a conscious effort to do this. It is most of the time an added chore to our busy day and we usually feel that there is no time to do this. But, like Grizabella, they will someday see their last street lamp flicker out and someone will take their place.

Sometimes just by looking back at some of the most primitive cultures when the elderly were revered and considered wise, we can learn more about who we have become as a 7society. Truly it is not that simple but it is something to ponder. Having dealt with so many deaths and families, I have seen how it can become just a matter of fact and just part of the big picture. It is ok to be wise and respected and it is ok to look up to your elders to see where they have come from and what they have gone through in their life. But more importantly, it is ok to be totally with a person who is dying and give them the dignity of listening to them. We will have plenty of time to speak later. This should be their time and anything we want to say to them, they already know and it will not matter soon.

We do this all the time with illness, elderly and dying. We are too caught up in the me, me, me, syndrome to experience the most amazing and miraculous moment in anyone's life unless it is a tragedy. Death.

ACKNOWLEDGMENTS

I want to acknowledge everyone who has ever made a difference in my life. From my parents and grandparents to my teachers and mentors who are too many to name. I have been lucky enough to have met people from all walks of life. Some of the most influential or inspiring were the homeless, dying, the disabled, and the teenagers and young people I have met all over the world. I understand the notion that "the children will lead us." It has come true in recent times, with the school shootings. I have to say that I have learned more from this group of people about life and its beauty than all the teachers I have known combined. What they gave me was a gift, not a lesson. They gave of themselves. They exposed their souls with no pretenses.

This book is about life through the eyes of a Caregiver, but one who has spent his whole life knowing that as a human among humans we are all Caregivers. Just recently I attended the memorial service of a young man who committed suicide. It made me think back to all the suicides I have encountered in my life, and how each one has affected me so differently, yet most of them have been out of the pain that we may all have at one time or another and cannot see or acknowledge. I want to acknowledge the fact that they lived and shared and loved and the pain they had was so engulfing that it took over any sense of clarity they had and led them to that place I hope we all may never see. It does bother me to hear people say that they will go to Hell if they commit suicide. Really? I would like to know how they came to that conclusion. When I look back, I see the judgment we as human beings place on others, not knowing how devastating it is for others. I also see how this judgment sometimes is supposed to inflict pain. Where have we come from and where are we going?

As a Caregiver, I have to say it is the most difficult job with the least monetary rewards and yet the most emotional rewards in many cases. Ask any person who is a Caregiver (and there is no shortage of them from nurses to PCAs, from teachers to coaches) what they do it for. It isn't the money in most cases. Most of them will tell you what it is about in story form, as it is impossible to explain. That is what this book is about. In story form, I have let you into a place where I can explain why I do it. Yet, I still do not know all the whys.

I hope you take time to tell someone who is a Caregiver, thank you, and that includes the people who are serving this country in the armed forces who are caring for our safety and protecting our freedoms. All Caregivers give something up and give of themselves unselfishly. That is admirable and something to be acknowledged. We need to begin the process of honoring this community. Caregivers come from every walk of life, from every corner of the earth. They are Black, White, Asian, Muslim, Jewish, and everything in between. There is no room for prejudices, racism, or politics yet it happens. Ask someone like Nate with CP who must rely on someone for everything in his life or Stephen Hawking, if you want to compare intelligence vs. disability. They will tell you the same thing. We are all equal. Our situations are different. That should not be judged.

I want to acknowledge you for reading this book. It is a sensitive subject for me and so many, but we all will be affected by the situations that could throw us into the stages where we need someone to help us live with dignity. These include old age, accidents or illness. They will all lead us there.

I am sad to finish this book that is never finished. I have been working and writing and editing since 1992. Twenty-five years of new experiences and side journeys from the main journey, my life as a Caregiver. I hope you have enjoyed reading this book. It is a very personal gift from me to you.

AUTHOR BIOGRAPHY

As a Caregiver, I have experienced many different scenarios of caregiving. As a young boy, I protected a friend with Down Syndrome from bullying daily. I volunteered to help with kids with disabilities in a youth group called STAR and was a US delegate to the Canadian National 4-H Convention. I went to RISD Art School High School program for six years and experienced College for 4 years with no degree. In 1969 I was founder and first director of Camp Happyness and was nominated for the Outstanding Young Men of America Award at Twenty. In 1970 I lived in Brazil and created several programs in the agricultural community in the rural farm area on an IFYE exchange. I was a house worker for a group home in Massachusetts. I worked with a camp for kids with Cancer as a photographer. I was a freelance photographer since my twenties and worked in retail and theater in NYC and was a Visual Display Artist for Bloomingdales, Victory Shirt Co, and many clothing and stationery stores. I worked with the homeless and substance abuse programs and HIV/AIDS Peer Education coordinator in Yonkers. I volunteered at Camp VIVA for families affected by HIV. I was a truck Driver, mill worker, and sales rep. On the board of the Stamford Arts Society and worked as an Educational Technician for several schools in Vermont for twenty-two years. I served on the Community Justice Center Board since 2014 and was Retail Manager for the Non-profit called ReSource. I now work with the mental health agency and have been a PCA for one young man for twenty plus years. My next goal is to continue restoring the 1900 vintage 16 room Victorian and turn it into a respite place for people with TBI. My mission in life is to enjoy it, learn from it, and leave it better than when I got here.

NOTES, QUOTES AND "AH-HA"'S

I would like to offer you a place in this book where you can write notes, quotes and some of the ah-ha moments you have experienced that this book may have sparked as a Caregiver, one being cared for or a bystander and a place to critique what you have read. It is called Notes, Quotes and Ah-ha's and is at the end of the book.

_____

_____

_____

_____

_____

_____

_____

_____

_____

_____

_____

_____

I would like to leave you with one last gift. This is a poem, public domain, which you might find interesting. I had this poem on my door and for many years and would read it before I left the house. It was a road map to where I am today and is one of the most profound poems I have known. It originally was not a poem, but a sermon. In 1971 it was an album by Les Crane with music by Broadway composer Fred Werner with the concept and various lyrics by David C. Wilson, and was a spoken word album. I hope it does for you what it has done for me. Peace.

Desiderata
(Latin for desired things)

Go placidly amid the noise and the haste and remember what peace there may be in silence. As far as possible, without surrender, be on good terms with all persons.

Speak your truth quietly and clearly; and listen to others, even to the dull and the ignorant; they too have their story.

Avoid loud and aggressive persons; they are vexatious to the spirit. If you compare yourself with others, you may become vain or bitter, for always there will be greater and lesser persons than yourself.

Enjoy your achievements as well as your plans. Keep interested in your own career, however humble; it is a real possession in the changing fortunes of time.

Exercise caution in your business affairs, for the world is full of trickery. But let this not blind you to what virtue there is; many persons strive for high ideals, and everywhere life is full of heroism.

*Be yourself. Especially, do not feign affection. Neither
be cynical about love; for in the face of all aridity and
disenchantment it is as perennial as the grass.*

*Take kindly the counsel of the years, gracefully
surrendering the things of youth.*

*Nurture strength of spirit to shield you in sudden misfortune.
But do not distress yourself with dark imaginings.
Many fears are born of fatigue and loneliness.*

*Beyond a wholesome discipline, be gentle with yourself.
You are a child of the universe, no less than the trees
and the stars; you have a right to be here.*

*And whether or not it is clear to you, no doubt the universe is unfolding
as it should. Therefore, be at peace with God, whatever you conceive Him
to be. And whatever your labors and aspirations, in the noisy confusion
of life, keep peace in your soul. With all its sham, drudgery and broken
dreams, it is still a beautiful world. Be cheerful. Strive to be happy.*

Desiderata by Max Ehrmann. 1927

If you are afraid you may not be complete with a person who is dying, think of it as though your phone battery is low and you say you are going to say good-bye to be complete. Because if the phone turns off in the middle of a conversation you will be complete.

Good-Bye.

Now I am complete.